Odyssey Now

The Old Ships

I have seen old ships sail like swans asleep
Beyond the village which men still call Tyre,
With leaden age o'er cargoed, dipping deep
For Famagusta and the hidden sun
That rings black Cyprus with a lake of fire;
And all those ships were certainly so old
Who knows how oft with squat and noisy gun,
Questing brown slaves or Syrian oranges,
The pirate Genoese
Hell-raked them till they rolled
Blood, water, fruit and corpses up the hold.
But now through friendly seas they softly run,
Painted the mid-sea blue or shore sea-green,
Still patterned with the vine and grapes in gold.

But I have seen
Pointing her shapely shadows from the dawn
An image tumbled on a rose-swept bay,
A drowsy ship of some yet older day;
And, wonder's breath indrawn,
Thought I – who knows – who knows – but in that same
(Fished up beyond Ææa, patched up new
– Stern painted brighter blue –)
That talkative, bald-headed seaman came
(Twelve patient comrades sweating at the oar)
From Troy's doom-crimson shore,
And with great lies about his wooden horse
Set the crew laughing, and forgot his course.

It was so old a ship – who knows, who knows?
– And yet so beautiful, I watched in vain
To see the mast burst open with a rose,
And the whole deck put on its leaves again.

James Elroy Flecker

Odyssey Now

Nicola Grove and Keith Park

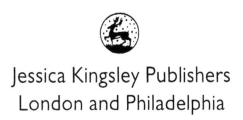

Jessica Kingsley Publishers
London and Philadelphia

Denotes individual pages that may be photocopied

First published in the United Kingdom in 1996
by Jessica Kingsley Publishers
116 Pentonville Road
London N1 9JB, UK
and
400 Market Street, Suite 400
Philadelphia, PA 19106, USA

www.jkp.com

Library of Congress Cataloging in Publication Data
Grove, Nicola, 1948-
Odyssey now / Nicola Grove and Keith Park.
p. cm.
Includes bibliographical references and index.
ISBN 1-85302-315-9 (pbk. : alk. paper)
1. Interactive video. 2. Homer. Odyssey. 3. Learning disabled-
-Education--Computer-assisted instruction. I. Park, Keith, 1952-
II. Title.
LB102.75.076   1996
371.3'3466--dc20   95-16493
CIP

British Library Cataloguing in Publication Data
Grove, Nicola
Odyssey Now
I. Title II. Park, Keith
371.904464

ISBN 978 1 85302 315 6

Contents

Acknowledgements

The ideas presented in this book have been stimulated through discussion with many people who have attended workshops, read first drafts, and provided helpful feedback. These include Jean Ware, Nick Peacey, Anna van der Gaag, Professor James Hogg, Barry Carpenter, Dawn Male and Jill Porter.

We would especially like to thank the following people for their continuing interest and support.

Olga Miller and Marcus Weisen from RNIB.

Nick Peacey and Gabriel Weissman, SENJIT.

All of those who piloted the programme, and sent us their comments: Helen Cockerill, staff and pupils of the Cheyne Centre; Ann Middleton, staff and pupils of Mapledown School; Gill Crawford, staff and pupils of Russett School; Bobbie Stormont, staff and pupils of Springfield School; Sally Slater, Woodford Lodge.

Participants at the RNIB *Odyssey Now* workshop, June 1994, who suggested adaptations of games to meet the needs of people with visual impairments: Margaret Ashford, Jane Jones, Alison Rampling, Patricia Ball, Wendy Cobb, Diane Quading, Farzana Naqui, Sarah Tooke, Lesley Billings, Anne Tucker, Carol Ouvry, Caroline Downs, Isobel Kelly, Lin Crane, Lynne Vaughan, Ann Veers, Sian Shaw, Ailsa Turner, Nicky Boden, Priya Stocks, Adam Ockelford and Derek Paravicini.

Original cover design by Gabriel Weissman, Applied and Fine Art.

The parachute game in *Charybdis* was suggested by Carol Wassall.

Some of the activities are derived from unattributed games used widely in classrooms. We acknowledge the inspiration afforded by others who have pioneered the use of drama with people who have profound and multiple learning disabilities.

Chapter 1

Introduction

Odyssey Now is a dramatisation of the story of Odysseus through a variety of interactive games, accompanied by music and pictorial slides. The title suggested itself because it is a recreation 'now' of the original and because the story is not only in words (n.o.w.). It is designed particularly to include people who have profound, severe or multiple learning disabilities; however, it can be used and adapted with any group of adults and children who have communication problems, in schools, colleges, homes and social education centres. It is also suitable for mixed ability groups, and could be used to promote integration between people with, and without, special needs. You don't need to know anything about the story to take part, nor have any particular skills in drama, music, story-telling or art. In fact, you should find that most of the activities are ones you are already doing in some form or other. The most important qualification for using the material is a willingness to try something new – we are aware from our own experience how easy it is to run out of energy and ideas when we are working with people who have very complex needs.

The Philosophy of Odyssey Now: Life Experiences for People with Profound and Multiple Learning Disabilities

Life experiences for people with profound and multiple learning disabilities can become very limited – as many parents, teachers and careworkers are aware. Art, music, drama and storytelling offer rich possibilities for stimulating the imagination, and extending experience (Mount 1995; Neelands 1992). But how can we best provide access to cultural experiences to people with very severe intellectual impairments? Bruner (1963, p.39) has suggested that 'any subject can

1

be taught effectively in some intellectually honest form to any child at any stage of development' (p.39). If he is right, then this statement should apply to everyone, whatever their level of disability. What might serve as the starting point?

A character in Oscar Wilde's *An Ideal Husband* remarks that he never goes to Strauss concerts 'because the music is always in German'. How necessary is verbal comprehension to the understanding of poetry and literature? We know that people with profound learning disabilities can enjoy music, so why not the music of words? Do we have to *comprehend* before we can *apprehend*? Does the 'meaning' of a poem or story have to be retrieved through a process of decoding individual words, or can it be grasped through a kind of atmosphere created through sound and vision? (See Webb 1992). We would like to suggest that all of us derive enjoyment from hearing music and poetry, and seeing pictures, often without being very sure what they 'mean'. Partly, this is a process of getting to know a work of art, so that we recognise familiar phrases, refrains, or visual patterns. As we get to know them better, so they take on meaning for us. This process of *apprehension* depends, we think, on repetition. Just as popular rhymes, jokes and tall stories are learned by frequent repetition, and passed from generation to generation, so snatches of poetry and prose, musical pieces and paintings can become recognisable by being repeatedly experienced in a structured context. Vygotsky (1978) proposed that 'human learning presupposes a specific social nature and a process by which children grow into the intellectual life of those around them' (p.89). Regardless of disability, we think that everyone has the capacity to come to know and enjoy the stories, art and music that form their 'cultural heritage'. The question is how to provide the access.

The Framework of Odyssey Now

With these considerations in mind, we have constructed a series of activities, based on Homer's story *The Odyssey*. It is one of the oldest stories in the Western world, and is particularly suitable for adaptation, because it has constantly been taken up and reworked with different audiences in mind. For example, a recent cartoon features Ulysses soaring through the galaxies in a spaceship; Tony Robinson has updated the stories for children's television in *Odysseus, the Greatest Hero of them All*. It's a strong and exciting adventure story, with many changes of atmosphere and mood, providing contrast and variety.

The ideas for activities arose out of group work which focused on interactive games. You will find that all the games in *Odyssey Now* are variations of things you are already doing. However enjoyable these are, when you play them as ends in themselves, they can become somewhat repetitive and meaningless. We started to experiment with presenting games in a narrative, multi-media context and thereby facilitating access to myths and stories for individuals with severe, or profound and multiple learning disabilities. Once we had begun, we found inspiration from many sources, including the *Galaxies* project (Consortium Team 1984) which is used successfully in many schools.

The aims of the programme are two-fold. First, to enhance the development of interactions with peers and staff members through a series of games rooted in one of the oldest stories of all. Second, to provide activities that we hope will stimulate teachers and care-workers to use their innate creativity in providing positive life experiences for the people with whom they work.

The activities have been chosen to meet certain criteria:

1. The skills demanded from the students should be *functional* in other contexts – i.e. they should be part of a repertoire of communicative behaviours which are useful in the individual's daily life. In the second section of the project, we suggest a framework for planning individual programmes to develop particular skills of communication; and a system of record-keeping for individuals and groups.

2. The activities should be easy to implement, easy to adapt, and cheap.

3. Each activity should relate coherently to the story line of the *Odyssey*. We approached the task by looking at the story, and abstracting key themes from each episode – then thought about how these themes could be translated into a game.

4. Additionally, we wanted to provide access to the aesthetic experience of art, music, and literature in a multi-sensory framework. These provide the 'background scenery', if you like, against which the story and the drama unfold. Rather than composing specific music, or designing specific pictures (both of which would of course be possible), we wanted students to experience what is already their enormously diverse, rich and exciting heritage. The criteria for choosing the slides and the music are highly personal, but reflect a wish to provide contrasts in atmosphere and style.

5. The activities should promote interactions between peers, at a group level as well as an individual level. Most of the work on communication with people with profound learning disabilities centres around building up one-to-one interactions, for obvious reasons. However, people also need to be helped to take an active part in the social group to which they belong. Games which involve people acting together may help to develop a sense of group identity.

6. Finally, the multi-dimensional nature of the project makes it particularly appropriate to delivering a broadly based curriculum (National or otherwise). The focus of the project is on developing personal–social skills, in the context of literature and drama, art and music. Many of the activities develop knowledge related to other areas, such as science, and there is ample scope to develop a range of associated activities. In the final section, some suggestions are given for relating the activities directly to attainment targets.

Drama in Odyssey Now

When we think of drama, it tends to be in terms of imaginative and symbolic behaviour, such as role-play in dramatic productions, where an event and the characters associated with it are re-presented in order to inspire feelings of 'pity and terror', or laughter and recognition, in the audience. How can we represent a story like the *Odyssey* to individuals who function cognitively at a level that is dominated by immediate actions and sensations; who neither use nor understand language, and whose ability to imagine is very difficult for us to determine? There are a number of possible ways to meet this challenge. In drama, there are many levels at which the action takes place. Gavin Bolton, a drama specialist in mainstream education, suggests that at a fundamental level drama is a kind of game, which functions at a level of mental representation concerned with actions *(enactive)* and images *(iconic)* which is 'not amenable to verbal, or other symbolic explicitness' (1986, p.61). This is an approachable way of thinking about drama for people who have profound learning disabilities. There is no requirement that they 'understand' a story, or imagine characters and events. The only requirement is participation in the playing of the game. This is in no way a trivialising of the experience. Bolton, quoting Huizinga, writes that 'Games demand order, and their elements, which also belong to aesthetics, are tension, poise, balance, contrast, variation, solution, resolution – the very elements of theatrical form' (p.64). Nor does the highly structured nature of game-playing preclude the development of the imagination. Vygotsky (1976) pointed out that 'every imaginative situation contains rules in a concealed form' (p.543): this principle can be reversed to state that 'every game with rules contains an imaginative situation in a concealed form'.

In fact, drama and games share features with all kinds of other social rituals that are important to us – dances, religious services and ceremonies, musical performances, and conversations. All involve interactions, which can be thought of as a kind of conversation, involving either individuals, or groups of people.

> An interaction is really…a dialogue between partners where each has the opportunity to communicate, and each has the obligation to respond. (Siegel-Causey and Guess 1989, p.10)

Often there is an alternation between the person acting as an autonomous, independent being, with the person as an interdependent being who is part of a group. In dances and playground games, individual pairs take solo roles while the group look on, then the whole group acts together. For example, in barn dances, everyone may dance in a circle, and then individual pairs dance, whilst the rest clap. In Greek drama, the Chorus and the individual characters alternate, just as they do in choral works like the *St. Matthew Passion*, or in a musical like *Joseph and the Technicolor Dreamcoat*. In *Odyssey Now*, the same principles are at work; people take it in turns to function as group members, and as individual 'actors' in the games. The activities are inherently dramatic – and you need no special skills as a drama teacher or therapist to play them.

How to Use this Project

The games and resources for the *Odyssey* story can be found in the next section. You may want to implement the programme simply as a self-contained leisure activity. However, if the programme is to be used as a way of developing communication skills, or as part of a curriculum, it is important to be clear about the relevance of the activities to your students, and to keep some kind of record of what happens in the sessions. The section on the **communication framework** sets out the model we have used as a basis for devising the games, so that each is genuinely purposeful. Each game is cross-referenced back to the communication model. The next section outlines the rationale underlying the **multi-sensory presentation** we have adopted. The section on **record-keeping** suggests a format for organising the programme, and relating it to the needs of the students with whom you are working. The final section suggests how *Odyssey Now* could be linked to the attainment targets in various subject areas of the **National Curriculum.**

The structure of *Odyssey Now* is based on the principles of a communication model which assumes that intention and understanding grow out of the repeated experience of the sequences and consequences of events. This is explained in detail in the section on communication. In other words, we are not assuming that the story will 'mean' anything to the students at the outset. Meaningful associations will develop as the games are played and re-played, and individuals come to anticipate what behaviours are expected in each episode. We have identified purposes for each activity which we believe are significant to the development of intentionality, and which may be functionally extended in everyday contexts. These include: eye gaze; exchanges and turn-taking; contingent vocalisation; gaining attention; anticipation; and elicitation of states of feeling which contrast with one another. Each activity is concerned with developing interactions between group members, rather than with staff members as such. Hence the role of staff members is to act as facilitators to promote interpersonal communication, and as 'scaffolders' to provide a meaningful structure to the storyline.

We have provided a mass of activities, and we're not suggesting you try to do all of them. The project, if used in full, could develop over the course of a school year, on a once-a-week basis – or you may wish to select only three episodes and develop them over a term. Some principles, however, are very important to maintain. First, a lot of repetition is called for. People learn to enjoy music, pictures, stories and games through having the opportunities to play them over and over again at leisure – and then to start to vary them a little. Many of the games we've suggested need working up to, and slow introductions. Secondly, we think it's vital to maintain consistent opening and closing sequences (**Setting off** and **Winding down**). At first, most of your session may consist of just these two activities. Then, gradually, they can be shortened, so that they take on the properties of a framework that marks the beginning and end of the session. This kind of framing occurs in communication (we have formalised ways of starting and ending conversations) and in stories *(Once upon a time…they lived happily ever after)*. We suggest, though, that you always leave at least five minutes for enjoying the pictures and music at the end of the session. Finally, never force people to take part in a game if they do not want to (this applies to staff as well as students!) The storyline is provided at the beginning of each episode, and could be read to the students, either before or after the setting off activity. Each activity has an introductory line or two, and we have indicated which words could be signed, by putting them in capitals.

Meeting Resistance

When we first suggested the idea of *Odyssey Now*, there were a lot of raised eyebrows. It might sound elitist and off-putting, and some people have argued that it is removed from the everyday needs of our students. We hope that we can persuade you that: (a) it's a brilliant story, which everyone can enjoy; (b) we need to nourish the imagination and emotions of students, as well as providing them with practical skills; and (c) it's fun to try something different. However, it is never a good idea to impose a programme on colleagues who feel reluctant and anxious about an approach which feels eccentric. Here are some suggestions which we have found helpful in winning people over:

- **Find allies.** Look for the people you work with who enjoy different kinds of music, films, theatre, books and art, and would like to share these experiences with people who have learning disabilities.

- **Plan the programme from the beginning with your staff team.** Involve them in choosing episodes, setting goals for individuals, choosing the music and slides. The section on record-keeping provides a step by step approach to implementation.

- **Discuss the principles behind the project.** Talk about the idea of using a storyline as a way of structuring communication activities, and making them fun. Draw parallels with the experience of young children, who can gain positively from all sorts of experience without understanding everything they see and hear.

- **Suggest integrating the project** with art and craft activities, and a visit to a gallery or concert where some of the music is being performed. The project can then be seen to contribute to goals of normalisation. If you are working in a school, the project can be seen as a way of effectively implementing the National Curriculum.

- **Stress that it is experimental.** You can change anything you like. You could take a different story, and use similar games.

Adaptations

Many of the activities involve movement, chasing and catching. People with severe physical disabilities, or who do not like to move from one place, can be pushed in wheelchairs, or pulled on blankets. Alternatively, slow the game right down by bringing the pursuer up to the person. Hold objects within their reach.

The Use of Physical Contact

We have all been made aware of the need to exercise caution about the use of touch between staff and clients. *Odyssey Now* involves a lot of physical contact, because of its importance as a channel of communication with people who have profound and multiple learning disabilities, so certain guidelines need to be followed:

- Be sensitive to a person's response – don't impose contact that they find difficult.

- Most of the activities involve the kind of contact that is normal and appropriate in everyday situations. For chase games and massage, prepare people by telling them what is going to happen, and showing them where they will be touched (demonstrate with another member of staff).

- Be aware of any reactions which seem extreme or inappropriate, such as arousal. If necessary, change the game – e.g. massage can be of hands only, catching can involve touch on the shoulder.

- Make the boundaries clear – ensure that each touch game has a clear beginning and end, and that people disengage, pause and come together before moving on to the next activity.

Slides and Music

The slides can be obtained by post from the National Gallery[1] – or you may want to explore what is available locally. The project provides opportunities for follow-up visits to galleries, where the students can recognise 'their' pictures on the walls. The music needs to be collected on to one or two tapes, and the numbers marked for ease of use. It's up to you how to use them – you could project the slide only at the beginning and end; only at the end, or all through. If you're only using it at the end, you might like to adopt a colour theme for each episode, using different-coloured light bulbs. Sometimes, when the atmosphere changes dramatically during one episode, we suggest changing the slide and music. Some episodes (e.g. 'Massage', 'Banquet') lend themselves to continuous slide projection, since they are not very active.

Finally, these activities are not set in stone! We think there is a great fund of creativity amongst people who work in this field, which sometimes gets eroded by the sheer hard slog of day-to-day caring and teaching. Feel free to adapt, change the sequence, or leave things out – but do keep a note of what happens! We would really like to know about games which work, new games, and games which fail completely.[2]

---

1   National Gallery, Trafalgar Square, London WC2N 5DN. Tel. 0171-839 3321.
2   Nicola Grove and Keith Park can be contacted in writing c/o Jessica Kingsley Publishers, 116 Pentonville Road, London N1 9JB.

Chapter 2

Activities

Summary of Activities

SETTING OFF	How Odysseus and his companions begin each adventure.
WINDING DOWN	How they end each adventure.
CYCLOPS	How they escape from a one-eyed man-eating giant.
CIRCE	How they are blown off course and enchanted by a witch.
HADES	How they visit the underworld to find answers to their questions.
SIRENS	How their way is barred by dangerous obstacles.
CALYPSO	How they are seduced from their path by a beautiful nymph.
NAUSICAA	How their ship is wrecked, and they find food and shelter.
ITHACA	How they return home and do battle with their enemies.

List of Resources

All activities	Tape recorder; slide projector; lamp with different coloured bulbs (optional).
CYCLOPS	Torch; balls – light plastic or newspaper; sheepskin (optional); wedges; tables; chairs.
CIRCE	Bag made out of a large piece of cloth or blanket, tied with string; blanket/parachute; large ball; strong-smelling plants.
HADES	Torches; blanket.
SIRENS	Wedges; tables; parachute.
CALYPSO	Massage oils, brushes, etc.; parachute or blanket; fan, water spray, seaweed.
NAUSICAA	Wedges, tables, chairs; musical instruments, waterspray; cloth or blanket; preferred foods.
ITHACA	Bag with disguises; gold crown; mirrors; bean bags, wedges, large ball; water pistols, cushions, bell; long strips of cloth or crepe paper.
Suggested slides:	(National Gallery slide numbers in brackets):
CYCLOPS	Turner: *Ulysses deriding Polyphemus* (508)
CIRCE	Botticelli: *Venus and Mars* (915)
HADES	Rembrandt: *Interior* (3214) or Turner: *Death on a Pale Horse* (Turner Gallery)
SIRENS	Cezanne: *Bathers* (6359)

CALYPSO	Velázquez: *Rokeby Venus* (2057)
NAUSICAA	Turner: *Calais Pier* (472)
	Melendez: *Still Life with Oranges* (6505)
ITHACA	Giordano: *Perseus turning Phineas into stone* (6487)
	Pintoricchio: *Scenes from the Odyssey* (911)

The storylines which are included in each episode are provided as a background. If you wish to tell the story as part of the activity, the language may need to be modified to suit the needs of the group.

Capital letters are used to denote manual signs which can be included in the introduction to the game (for example, CRASH, EAT, STRONG).

Setting Off

Everyone sits in two parallel lines, behind each other. A leader (Odysseus) sits in front. Move backward and forward in unison, making rowing movements. After a few moments, Odysseus shouts 'STOP'.

The story	Odysseus and his friends are setting sail in their boat on the long journey home. They will have many adventures, at sea, and on the islands they visit. After each adventure, they set off again.
Themes	Beginnings and endings.

Music suggestions	Sea shanties.
	Paul Robeson – 'Shenandoah'.
	Rod Stewart – 'Sailing'.
	Mendelssohn – *Fingal's Cave*.
	Britten – *Sea Symphony*.

Introduction	'We're going in a BOAT. We're going on a long journey HOME.'
Purposes	*Intentional movement. Group awareness and interaction. Physical co-ordination. Discriminative reaction to word/sign. Understand word/sign for STOP. Understand that the session is beginning.*

Variations

Sit/stand in a circle, and hold a blue cloth or parachute. Wave it up and down to represent the sea. Bring it up high, and down over everyone's heads. Now you're under the sea – what will happen when you emerge?

More able students can act as leaders, and can speed the movement up, slow it down, or beat a drum to give the rhythm (Remember the film of *Ben Hur*?).

Students who need a quieter or less active opening could spend a short time looking at the picture, and listening to the music for the relevant episode.

This activity (or another that you might think of) can act as the opening sequence each week, to orientate the students to the session. You can shorten it progressively, so that it becomes no more than a quick device.

Winding Down

Bring the group together, in comfortable relaxed positions. Project the appropriate picture, and put on the music, which you used for the episode. Spend five minutes just looking and listening. Try always to make sure that you leave enough time for this activity. You can use this period of time for jotting down notes about what happened in the session.

Introduction	We've FINISHED our journey for today. TIME to RELAX. LISTEN to the MUSIC. LOOK at the PICTURE.
Purposes	*Understand that the session is ending. Calm down after activities. Enjoy the picture and the music.*

Episode 1. Cyclops

The story

Odysseus and his companions land on the island of the Cyclops, a huge giant, with only one eye. They go into a dark cave, where the Cyclops keeps his sheep. He comes home and traps them in the cave. He wants to eat them all. Odysseus tricks the Cyclops. He gives him wine to drink, and when the giant has fallen asleep, makes him blind by driving a stick into his one eye. In the morning, the Cyclops has to let his sheep out of the cave. Odysseus tricks him again. Each sailor gets underneath a sheep, and holds onto its belly. The sheep go out of the cave, and the Cyclops feels them as they go past. Of course, he does not know the men are there. They get to their boat and get ready to sail away. Odysseus teases the giant, and shouts at him. The Cyclops is furiously angry, and throws huge rocks at the ship, but Odysseus and his friends escape safely.

Themes

Danger. Secrecy. Fear. Escape. Exultation.

Music suggestions	Mussorgsky – 'Gnomus' (from *Pictures from an Exhibition*).
	Liszt – *Mazeppa*.
	any film score you can find with music to accompany a chase, e.g. *Jaws*.
	Philip Glass – *Koyaanisqatsi*.
Slide suggestions	Turner – *Ulysses Deriding Polyphemus* (National Gallery).
	any terrifying picture of a giant, or one-eyed creature (try Picasso).
Colour	Green.

Smell	Cedar or pine aromatic oil – something astringent.
Resources	Torch, Balls (plastic or newspaper). Sheepskin (optional). Wedges, tables, chairs.

1. Who's for Dinner

Everyone sits in a circle. A member of staff is the Cyclops, and begins to walk around the inside, rhythmically chanting, for example, 'Fee fi foh fum, look out dinner, here I come.' or 'I want *(name)* for my lunch. I hate the taste but I love the crunch'.

On the final word, the Cyclops shines the torch on the victim, and grabs him/her for dinner. Students can then take turns to act as the Cyclops.

Introduction	We've left the boat. We're on an island. LOOK! There's a giant.
Purposes	*Anticipation. Elicit thrill, fear, excitement. Directed gaze. Joint attention. Interaction. Negation.*

Variations

Call the name of the person you are going to eat.

Walk around the outside of the circle, in time to the music, firmly placing your hand on the shoulder of each person in turn, and pretending to eat them.

2. One Eye

With the room as dark as possible, the 'Cyclops' is in the middle of the floor with a torch (the one eye) beside him/her. The Cyclops says, 'If I shine my LIGHT on you, you're DEAD!' The others sit in a circle, and one by one, try to creep up and take the torch, without making a sound. If a noise is heard, the Cyclops picks up the torch, shines it in the direction of the noise, and calls out the person's name/says 'NO! GO back'. The person who has been spotted goes back to the starting line. The one who gets the torch becomes the Cyclops. Encourage people to look, turn their heads or move towards the light source.

Introduction	LOOK! There's the giant. If he sees us, we're DEAD. We need to get his LIGHT. Ssh. Don't let him hear you.
Purposes	*Elicit feelings of excitement, apprehension, humour. Goal-directed movement. Co-ordination. Anticipation. Turn-taking. Name recognition. Negation.*

Variation

Once people can do this in a circle, try approaching in a group from the end of the room ('Grandmother's Footsteps').

Visual impairment

Put bells around the torch and rattle them softly to show where it is. If a visually impaired person is the Cyclops, put the torch on rustly material. Provide a running commentary.

3. Sheep Escape

Make a 'cave' area with wedges, tables, chairs, with an entrance wide enough for the Cyclops to sit in, and a person to get past. Make the room dark, and/or blindfold the Cyclops. People must go past him or her in turn, crawling if possible. The Cyclops feels each person, and tries to say who it is. If the guess is wrong, the person escapes. If they are right, that person becomes the Cyclops. Have a staff member sit opposite the cave, beckoning people to come to him or her.

(If you have a sheepskin, it can be put on by the escapee, to make the Cyclops' job more difficult.)

Introduction	LOOK, THERE's the giant. You must CREEP past him. He will touch you as you go. Will he KNOW your NAME?

Purposes	*Elicit feelings of excitement, apprehension, humour. Name recognition. Interaction through reach, touch. Turn-taking.*

4. Boulder Escape

One or more people are the Cyclops, in the middle of the room with a supply of rocks (light plastic balls, or screwed-up newspaper). A staff member stands at the other end of the room, where the 'boat' is. The task is to get from one end of the room to the other without getting hit. Winners can become Cyclops.

Introduction	LOOK, THERE's the giant. Get to the boat as fast as you can. RUN. Be CAREFUL – he's THROWing rocks at us.
Purposes	*Elicit feelings of excitement, apprehension, humour. Co-ordination. Anticipation. Turn-taking.*

Visual impairment

Sailors should make a continuous noise as they run, so that a visually impaired Cyclops can aim in their direction. Provide a commentary to say who has been hit, and who has escaped.

When you get to the 'boat' encourage the crew to wave and jeer at the giant, shouting things like 'Hooray', 'You can't get us now', 'Goodbye sucker'. The Cyclops can retaliate with 'I'll get you next time. Just you wait', etc. as the sailors row away.

Episode 2. Circe

The story

Odysseus and his crew have been staying with Aeolus, the god of winds. He gives them a large bag, and tells them not to open it until they are near home. Odysseus' friends want to know what is in the bag, so they open it. A great stormy wind rushes out and blows them to Circe's island. Circe is a witch and has magic powers; she casts a spell over some of the sailors and turns them into pigs. Odysseus finds a magic herb (moly) to break the spell, and change them back into men again. Then they set off again on their journey.

Themes

Being blown off course. Capture. Enthralment. Escape.

Music suggestions	Verdi – 'Slaves Chorus' from *Nabucco*.
	Beethoven – 'Prisoners' Chorus' from *Fidelio*.
	Janacek – *Sinfonietta*.
	Tria Bulgarca – *Mystère du Voix Bulgare*.
	Cream – *Strange Brew*.
Slide suggestion	Botticelli – *Venus and Mars*.
Colour	Orange.
Smell	Sandalwood.
Resources	A large, loose 'bag' made from a piece of cloth by bringing the corners together, and tying a string around them. Blanket/parachute. Large ball. Strong-smelling plants.

1. Aeolus

Everyone sits in a circle. A staff member acts as Aeolus, and arrives with the bag.

Introduction	I'm GIVING you a present to help you on your journey, but you must NOT OPEN it yet. It's got something special inside it. Just put it somewhere safe until you are nearly home.

Put on the music, and play 'pass the parcel' with the bag. When the music stops, the person who is holding the bag is asked if they want to open it. Staff members should take different roles, some saying 'Oh, go on, it'll be OK, I want to know what's inside', etc., while others advise against it. Encourage people to speculate about what is inside. If they indicate 'no' the music is put on again, and the bag handed on. Do this two or three times, and if everyone is saying no, get a staff member to say yes.

Open the bag, and then create a huge gust of wind by waving the cloth up and down. Get knocked over by it. Exclaim 'My goodness, it's a really strong WIND what's going to happen now?'

Purposes	*Turn-taking – offering and taking. Negation. Comments and Question. Anticipation.*

2. Blown Away

Make Circe's island at one end of the room with a large mat. One person sits on a blanket, and is pulled to an 'island'. The others act as the wind, blowing him or her, with hands, fans and cloths. Each person can take it in turn.

Purposes	*Joint attention. Vocalisation. Goal-directed behaviour. Anticipation. Experiencing/tolerating changes.*

Variations

Everyone sits in a circle. Two people in the middle hold a blanket and wave it up and down, creating a draught. They repeat 'The wind is coming, it's coming for you' three times, increasing the volume, until they finally say 'It's coming for [name]' then drop the blanket over a person's head and let it go. Encourage people to push the blanket off, and indicate who should take a turn next.

Use hands, fans, cloth to move a large light ball around the room. One team can try and blow it in one direction, the others try to get it to their side.

Visual impairment

Have wind chimes tinkling to indicate where the island is. Ask people to indicate its direction, as you pull them along on the blanket. The sound stops when the island is reached.

3. Circe

When everyone has arrived on the mat, have a staff member stand to one side, looking witch-like. He or she creates a 'pen' area with chairs:

Introduction	Circe says: 'You've left your boat. You're on my island. I'm CIRCE. I'm a witch. Don't let me CATCH you. If I do you must come into my prison. Only your leader can set you free.'

Circe is 'it' and everyone who is touched by her has to go to the 'pen' at one end of the room. Another person is Odysseus, and can release them by touching them. People can take it in turns to be Circe, and see who can capture the most.

Purposes	*Interaction through touch and chase. Anticipation. Goal-directed behaviour. Elicit feelings of fear, enjoyment, excitement.*

Variations

Instead of a 'pen' students must stand still where they are caught until released.

Visual impairment

Circe could wear a witch's hat and long nails which can be felt. Provide a commentary about who has been caught, and who is free.

4. Moly

Use two or three strong smelling plants like lavender, spring onion, mint (moly was a type of wild garlic, which you could also use). Present the smells to a person (Odysseus) who must choose which one he or she wants to be the moly. One or two people are captured by Circe and stand in frozen positions. Odysseus touches them with the moly to release them.

Purposes   *Identifying scents. Interaction through touch.*
Anticipation.Goal-directed behaviour.

Variations

Blindfold Odysseus, and let him/her smell one of the plants. He or she must identify it out of the three before using it to release the captives.

'Hide' the plant around the room. Help Odysseus to hunt for it (Draw a picture to show what it looks like; hide contrasting vegetables, like carrots, potatoes.) Can he or she find the moly? Introduce a time limit – the captives will explode if you don't get there in time.

Episode 3. Hades

The story	Odysseus visits the entrance to Hades, a place of ghosts, to ask if they know what will happen to him, and when he will get home. He calls up the ghosts by killing two sheep – the souls of the dead come in their multitudes to drink the blood from the pit. Among them are former friends and the ghost of his own mother.
Themes	The traditional associations of Hallowe'en. Uncertainty, fear and strangeness. Thresholds. Transformations. Questions about the future.

Music suggestions	Hitchcock-type film music.
	Bartok – 'Adagio' (*Music for Strings, Percussion and Celeste*).
	Webern – *Six pieces for Large Orchestra* (Nos. 1, 4).
	Gorecki's *Third Symphony*.
	'Song of the Sibyl' (from the *Livre Vermeilh de Montserrat*).
	Pentangle – 'Lyke-Wake Dirge' (on the album *Basket of Light*).
Slide suggestions	Rembrandt: *Interior*.
	Turner: *Death on a Pale Horse* (Turner Gallery).
Colour	Black.
Smell	Earth or mould (bring in a compost bucket).
Resources	Torches. Blanket.

1. Lights and Shadows

Make sure the room is dark, or very dim.

Introduction 'We've come to a strange, dark place. WHO is HERE? WHAT can they TELL us?

Use torches to explore how we change into shadows. First allow people to get used to the torches – pass them round, switch them on and off, shine them at people. Keep asking questions like: 'Who is it? Oh, it's you!'

1. Then experiment with 'odd faces'. Shine a powerful torch up into your mouth, and your face becomes translucent. At a particular angle under your chin, your face looks very strange. Make some spooky noises as you do so.

2. Hold the torch pointing upright at the ceiling. Very slowly, bring your hand down over it, encouraging people to look up at the ceiling as you do so. It looks as though a giant hand is moving to engulf everyone.

3. Put the torch, or a strong light, behind a screen. Move hands in front of it to make shadow plays. Prompt different individuals to go behind the screen, for others to guess who it is. Two people can 'meet' on the screen.

Purposes *Directed gaze. Intentional movement, and sound making. Experiencing noticing – tolerating changes. Elicit thrill, fear, uncertainty.*

NB Some of these games can actually be quite unsettling, and may need to be developed very gradually and interspersed with a lot of reassurance. They are included because the excitement of being scared, in a safe environment, is fun and a valuable dramatic experience.

2. Ghost Train

Create a ghostly environment to pass through. Make twittering, rustling, humming sounds to represent the presence of the shades. Trail 'cobwebs' over hands and faces. Have a feelie bag of objects and textures – a 'dead man's hand' (water in a rubber glove), blood (ketchup), a sailor's eye (peeled grape, or satsuma with a hole in it), entrails (cold spaghetti). You must pass through these ordeals before getting to ask your questions. Once the students are familiar with the activities, they can be the ones to create the environment, and make the staff go through the ordeals.

Purposes   *Differentiating experiences through touch. Tolerating changes. Elicit thrill, uncertainty, excitement.*

3. Who Is in the Pit?

Each person takes it in turn to sit in the middle of the circle, under a sheet. The group chants 'Who is in the pit? Who is in the pit?', and gradually the sheet is pulled off, to cries of 'It's [name]'. Encourage the person to reach out towards another individual, who becomes the next 'soul in the middle'.

Purposes   *Understanding names. Interaction through reaching. Elicit uncertainty, fear and recognition. Turn-taking: initiation and response.*

Variations

Prompt the person in the middle to pull the sheet off him/herself. Prompt others to go and pull the sheet off, and greet the person by touching, shaking hands, making eye contact.

4. Questions

Take it in turns to point the torch at a person, and ask him or her a question.

These can range from very simple, standard questions, with a prompted yes/no response. For people with very limited understanding of speech or sign, the question and answer can be kept the same each time the game is played; e.g. 'Is your name…' 'Would you like a tickle/hug/song?' (make sure you give it to them immediately).

At the other extreme, students with good verbal or sign comprehension can be asked more demanding, open-ended 'fortune-telling' questions, such as: 'Do you think it will rain tomorrow?', 'Will Liverpool win the cup?', 'Do you think my boyfriend will ring me this evening?'

Purposes   *Turn-taking. Understanding and responding to question routines – yes and no. Asking questions.*

Variations

Take it in turns to spin the torch in the centre of the circle, and see who it points to.

Encourage those who can to think of some questions – even very simple ones like 'What's your name?'.

Combine this game with 'Who is in the pit?' by having the person under the sheet answer the questions (you may have to take the sheet off first!).

5. In the Light of Day

Because Hades is such an unsettling place, it is important to return to normal life!

Introduction   It's time to leave this DARK place, and return to the LIGHT of DAY.

Go back through the ghost train, or create a tunnel through which people can pass by putting a parachute over tables. Bring each person out in turn and welcome them back to the land of the living. Bring the lights up slowly and use a tape such as dawn chorus, sea sounds, bells or gentle music for reassurance.

Episode 4. Sirens

The story

Odysseus and his friends meet some dangerous obstacles which they have to get round safely. The first is the clashing rocks. You must get between them before they squash you. The next is Scylla ('Skee-la) a monster with six heads, and three rows of teeth. She lives in a cave, and snatches men off each boat that goes past. Then she eats them. Charybdis (Car-'ib-dis) is a whirlpool – water that goes round and round very fast, which sucks boats into the middle. The Sirens are girls with the most beautiful voices in the world, who lure sailors to death – their island is covered with skeletons and withered skin.

There are four main activities: one or two can be chosen each time.

Themes

Obstacles. Danger. Enchantment.

Music suggestions	Elgar – 'Where corals lie' (*Sea Pictures*).
	Saint-Saëns –'Fishes' (*Carnival of the Animals*).
	Verdi – 'Un di felice' (*La Traviata*).
	Joan Armatrading – 'Love and Affection'.
Slide suggestion	Cézanne: *Bathers.*
Colour	Blue.
Smell	Seaweed (get a mound from the seaside, keep it in salt water).
Resources	Wedges, tables, skipping ropes.

1. Clashing Rocks

Two staff members act as 'rocks', by holding wedges in front of them, and moving slowly towards each other until they bump. Demonstrate this a few times. The task is to get between the two opposing rocks without being squashed. If you are caught, you can become a rock. 'Rocks' have to watch each other, co-ordinate their movements and interact physically; 'sailors' have to judge when to move, watch the 'rocks' and interact physically.

Introduction	LOOK out! In front of us are two great rocks. We have to get between them before they squash us!
Purposes	*Directed gaze. Intentional movement. Co-ordination. Adapting behaviour to negotiate an obstacle. Interaction. Anticipation. Elicit feelings of fear, humour, excitement.*

Visual impairment

Attach something which makes a sound to the rocks. If visually impaired people are acting as the rocks, pass through slowly, making a continuous noise. Encourage people to call out when caught, or clash cymbals. Vary the game – the task is to listen for the moving rocks, and avoid them. Provide a commentary to let people know what is happening.

2. Scylla

Erect a screen with tables/wedges. One person is Scylla, and hides behind it. Each sailor in turn must creep past the rock to safety. Every so often, she reaches out her long arm, grabs someone and 'eats' them. Demonstrate first with staff members. Keep the uncertainty level up by only capturing one or two people.

Introduction	LOOK out! Behind this rock is a sea monster. We have to get past without her catching us.

| Purposes | *Directed gaze. Intentional movement. Co-ordination. Interaction. Anticipation. Object permanence – disappearance and re-appearance. Elicit feelings of fear, humour, excitement. Interaction through reach and touch.* |

Visual impairment

Scylla signals her intentions by making a sound, increasing in volume just before she pounces. Provide a commentary.

3. Charybdis

Put a person in the middle of a parachute, then walk round and round, holding onto the edge, until the person is wrapped up. Then reverse direction, walking round and outwards, so that the person is spun out of the parachute.

| Introduction | LOOK out! In front of us the SEA spins ROUND and ROUND. If we are caught in it, we'll drown! |
| Purposes | *Directed gaze. Intentional movement. Co-ordination. Interaction. Anticipation. Elicit feelings of fear, humour, excitement.* |

Variations

Half the group act as Charybdis and form a circle. Capture people in wheelchairs and spin them round.

Move around one person in the middle, gradually getting closer and closer, until the person is squashed.

In the actual story, Odysseus has to move between Scylla and Charybdis. Once the group are familiar enough with the games, you can run them simultaneously. The group would then move slowly in a line between the two dangers, with two people being caught from each direction.

4. Sirens

This activity is essentially a dance, similar to 'Nuts in May', of approach and withdrawal. Split the group into unequal numbers of Sailors (more) and Sirens (less), standing in two parallel lines opposite each other. Switch on the tape recorder, and gradually bring up the sound of the music.

Introduction	LOOK out! In front of us are sirens (mime sexy contours). They want us to GO to them. But if we go, they will KILL us. LISTEN, can you hear them SINGING?

In time to the music, the Sirens move forward, holding hands, towards the Sailors. The Sailors move back as they advance. Then the Sirens move back, and the Sailors move forward. Once the group have mastered this basic movement, the sirens huddle together, and choose a Sailor. They then try to pull him/her across to their side of the room. The two friends on either side of the Sailor try to keep him/her with them. You will have to rig it at first so that the two sides become more equal. Alternate the choosing part of the dance with forward and backward movement.

Purposes	*Directed gaze. Intentional movement. Co-ordination. Group awareness and interaction. Anticipation. Elicit feelings of fear, humour, excitement.*

Variations

Another way of playing this is for the Sirens to keep doing their basic movement, being encouraged to reach towards the Sailors. One Sailor becomes Odysseus, and tries to leave his group to go to the Sirens. His friends have to stop him by holding on to him, saying 'No'.

If the group is big enough, it's fun to divide into girls and boys to play this.

Visual impairment

Join Sailors to Sirens with thick elastic ropes of tights or lycra. The Sirens haul in the Sailors, and let them go, in time to the music. Sirens call out 'I'm coming to get you', and say the name of the person they are aiming for.

Sirens sing, or make enticing sounds (jingling anklets). Sailors listen to tell if they are in the line of fire, and try to avoid them. Provide a commentary.

Episode 5. Calypso

| The story | The sailors land on Calypso's luxurious island. She keeps them there for several years. Eventually, she is persuaded to let them go and they set off again, leaving Calypso behind, in tears. |

| Themes | Enthralment. Sensuality. Parting. |

Music suggestions	Gershwin – 'Summertime' (*Porgy and Bess*).
	Mood music: *Paradise Island* (one of the tapes you can get with sea sounds and tropical noises).
	Jean-Michel Jarre e.g. *Oxygène*.
	Alain Stivell – *Renaissance of the Celtic Harp*.
For Leaving You	B.B. King – 'The Thrill is Gone'.
	John Mayall – 'Somebody Broke Your Wings'.
	'Jamaica Farewell'.
	Suzanne Vega – 'Calypso'.
	Shirley Collins – 'Our Captain Cried'.
	Edith Piaf – 'Ne me quitte pas'.
	Purcell – 'Dido's Farewell' (*Dido and Aeneas*).
Slide suggestion	Velázquez: *Rokeby Venus*.
Colour	Red.
Smell	Coconut massage oil. Suntan lotion-type smells.
Resources	Massage oils, brushes etc. Parachute or blanket.

1. Massage

Varieties of hand, foot, scalp massage; hairbrushing etc. Notes can be kept regarding individual preferences. Encourage individuals to extend a hand for more stroking; pick up objects and give them to you. Accompany with music; try to use one scent only.

Introduction	We've come to Calypso's island – we can all relax.
Purposes	*Relaxation. Enjoyment. Choice-making.*

2. Calypso Says…

One person is Calypso, stands in the middle of the circle, and gives commands to everyone else. He or she can either say or sign them, or perform actions that everyone else must copy. He or she can choose the next person to take his or her place.

Introduction	I am Calypso. YOU MUST do what I SAY.
Purposes	*Joint attention. Imitation. Vocalising/gesturing/signing. Group awareness and interaction. Commanding.*

3. Leaving You

Divide into pairs; one person does the going away, the other remains behind. The person who is leaving strokes down the other person's arms and hands very slowly, and then moves away, retaining fingertip contact so that hands are stretched out to one another. Repeat this action, moving further away each time. The atmosphere should be slow and sad. If movement away is too difficult, just end each time by turning your head and body away from the other person. It's obviously easier to do if a staff member is doing the leaving, since this is the more active part, but try to facilitate the activity so that the person with disabilities sometimes does the leaving.

Introduction	We have to GO now. We have to say GOODBYE to Calypso.

| Purposes | *Evoke awareness of another person. Feelings of sadness and loss. Turn-taking – greeting and parting. Interaction through touch.* |

Variations

If it is too difficult to pair off, sit in a circle, and take it in turns to be Calypso and Odysseus in the middle.

Make the activity into a group dance, by standing opposite each other in parallel lines. The front couple 'leave' one another, as described above, then peel off and move behind the lines till they get to the back. A second couple then become the pair to leave each other.

4. To Sea, To Sea

If a person can be lifted, place him/her in a blanket or the middle of the parachute and gently swing them to and fro. Others sit in a circle around. Hold a fan near the person's face; spray him/her gently with a water spray; wave seaweed under his/her nose).

| Introduction | We have to leave Calypso's island now, and go back to sea. |

| Purposes | *Relaxation. Enjoyment. Sensory experiences.* |

Episode 6. Nausicaa

The story

Odysseus leaves Calypso's island and is shipwrecked after a terrible storm. He swims to another island. There he meets Nausicaa (Nor-sic-'ay-a), who takes him to her father's palace where he receives food and drink. After dinner, he tells the stories of all his adventures so far.

Themes

Catastrophe. Danger. Safe havens. Hospitality. Storytelling.

Music suggestions	The Doors – 'Riders on the storm'.
	Beethoven – *Pastoral Symphony*.
	Elgar – *Sea Pictures*.
	Sibelius – *The Tempest*.
Slide suggestion	Turner: *Calais Pier*.
Colour	Blue.
Smell	Seaweed.
Resources	Wedges, cushions, etc. Musical instruments. Spray. Food.

I. The Storm

Form into a circle, sitting or standing. Pile wedges, cushions, polystyrene trays etc. into the middle, to act as the rocks. Pass round musical instruments.

Introduction

A storm is coming! Hear the thunder! (*noise of thunder*). Hear the wind! (*noise of wind; feel of wind*). Feel the rain! (*squirt water*).

Purposes

Anticipation. Discriminative reactions to sounds and tactile stimuli. Sound–meaning correspondence.

Variations

The group could split into thunder, wind and rain sections; make the noise when a leader (Odysseus) points to them.

2. The Wreck

Two people at a time run round the circle (or are pushed in wheelchairs) and then into the middle, where they fall onto the wedges, and knock them over. Everyone else chants: 'We're going to CRASH, we're going to CRASH'. Repeat till everyone has had a turn.

Introduction	'Oh no! we're going to CRASH on the rocks!'
Purposes	*Anticipation. Elicit fear, excitement and humour. Turn-taking. Understand, imitate, and/or produce word/sign CRASH.*

Variations

Encourage people to ask to take a turn; or have 'Odysseus' nominate who is going next.

3. Lifesaving

Designate an area of the room as an island space (you could put a yellow sheet there for sand). Four people hold each end of a parachute, blue sheet, or strip of cloth, and wave it up and down. Each individual must get to the island, by going under or over the cloth – crawling, walking, running, or being pushed. More able individuals might like to mime swimming.

Introduction	'We must SWIM to the island over THERE!'
Purposes	*Intentional movement towards a specified location. Adapting behaviour to negotiate an obstacle. Turn-taking.*

Variations

Introduce a shark to chase people to the island. Make a human chain from the beach to help others from the waves. 'Drown' people by catching them in the cloth if they aren't fast enough.

Visual impairment

Provide a track to the island which can be felt – e.g. sandpaper, imitation pineapples, wrappers of famous chocolate bars with desert island connotations. Put sand on the island so it is clear when they have reached it. Encourage people to get to the island by calling out encouragements – 'over here', 'yes, come on' etc. Chocolate awaits those who succeed.

4. Everybody Safe?

Ask one person to 'find' everyone in the group by name, by reaching out to them, pointing to, looking towards, or touching them. Encourage the rest of the group to respond by looking and extending a hand. Finish by all holding hands in a circle.

Introduction	'Are we all safe? Is EVERYONE HERE?'
Purposes	*Recognising and responding to friends.* *Turn-taking – greeting. Name recognition.* *Interaction through reach and touch.*

Variations

You could have a 'register' of photos that the concerned leader (Odysseus) must check through to make sure all his crew are safely landed.

Visual impairment

Everyone wears a tactile badge, with a matching badge on aboard. At the very beginning of the session, Odysseus checks the register to see that everyone is here. He must check again by matching the badges worn by the sailors, to the ones on the board.

5. Banquet

This activity aims to introduce different food and drink in whatever way is appropriate. For example, if one person needs liquidised food, and another requires a vegetarian diet, use a blender to make carrot juice; try home-made ice-cream, new tastes, ethnic foods, etc. Keep notes concerning individual preferences. Encourage students to offer food to one another.

Purposes   *Choice-making. Taste experiences. Relaxation. Enjoyment.*

Change slide projection to Melendez: *Still Life with Oranges.*

Music suggestions	Lute or guitar music e.g. John Williams and Julian Bream – *Together.*
	Baroque music e.g. Telemann, Bach, Vivaldi.
Colour	Yellow.
Smell	Food smells or Citrus oils.
Resources	Preferred foods.

6. Storytelling

After the food, sit round in a semi-circle, facing a large cushion/bean-bag and introduce a story-telling session. Each person takes it in turn to sit on the cushion, and 'tell a story'. You can choose how to do this. It can be something that has actually happened, however small, or a joke, or it could be an opportunity to tell stories from *Odyssey Now* – what happened with the Cyclops; what happened in the wreck. The 'story' does not have to be an extended narrative; it can be one or two words or signs that refer to an event. People who cannot talk or sign can show photographs to the group (you could take pictures of the *Odyssey Now* sessions to use here). You can also programme a communication aid, such as an Introtalker, with some of the intro-ductory phrases – e.g. the Cyclops saying 'If I shine my light on you, you're dead!', and use these as a way of recalling the games.

Purposes   *Intentional and reciprocal communication.*
                        Turn-taking. Comments about an event.

Visual impairment

Use a sensory story board, with smells, and a tactile cue from each
episode – e.g. Circe's finger nails and moly; Calypso's coconut oil;
cold spaghetti from Hades. Go through them one by one, and pass
them round as a concrete reminder. Some people may be able to
identify the item, and indicate what they can remember.

Episode 7. Ithaca

The story	Odysseus finally arrives home. He enters his palace in disguise, recognised only by his dog, and his old nurse. The palace is full of men who have been pestering his wife to marry one of them, because they believe that Odysseus is dead. Odysseus sits quietly on the guest bench during their feasting, but then takes part in a competition to draw the enormous bow he left behind. Only he can do it – and in that moment he is recognised. His friends come to help him, and there is a great battle. At the end, the intruders are all dead, and Odysseus meets his wife Penelope. She tricked the men by promising that she would marry one of them when she had finished her weaving – only she unpicked the work every night, so it was never finished
Introduction	'At last! Our journey is over. We're HOME. But we've been away a long time. We'd better find out what's been happening here'.
Themes	Homecoming. Disguise. Danger. Conflict. Trial of strength. Reunion.

Music suggestions	Beethoven's Fifth and Third Symphonies (loud bits).
	Strauss – *Also sprach Zarathustra* (*2001* theme tune).
	Prokofiev – Fight scene from *Romeo and Juliet*.
	Mussorgsky – 'Great Gate of Kiev' (*Pictures at an Exhibition*).

Slide suggestion	Giordano: *Phineas and his Companions Turned to Stone.*
Colour	Purple.
Smell	Eucalyptus.
Resources	Bag with disguises. Gold crown. Mirrors. Bean bags. Wedges. Large ball. Water pistols. Cushions. Bell. Long strips of cloth/crêpe paper.

1. Disguise

Sit in a circle. One person goes and knocks on the door, and a member of staff enters, carrying a bag of disguises. He or she explains that while you have been away, other people have come to live in the house, so it's dangerous. You need to disguise yourselves. Have a bag of hats, scarves, funny noses, dark glasses etc. Include a gold crown. Experiment with putting them on, taking them off, putting them on each other. Look in mirrors. Who *are* these people?

Purposes   *Experience/tolerate/bring about change. Goal-directed behaviour. Turn-taking – giving and taking objects. Name recognition. Jokes.*

Variations

Have a staff member (later a student) sit in the middle of the circle. Each student puts something on to change the way he or she looks.

Blindfold a member of staff. He or she must touch a person in disguise (or not) and guess who it is. If he or she is right, that person gets the crown, and becomes Odysseus.

This activity can be an alternative to 'Who is the Strongest' – the person who chooses the crown becomes the King and gets to choose the teams in Activity 3.

Visual impairment

Use disguises which have sound attached, strong bright colours, and glittery things which catch the light. Use items that can be felt – moustaches, plastic ears and noses, half masks, hats with corks. Start by feeling a staff member, then feeling the item, then putting it on the staff member. Allow people to explore these before putting them on themselves, as they may find it unsettling. Provide a commentary.

2. Who is the Strongest?

Practise lots of different trials of strength, depending on individual skills and preference: e.g. weight-lifting (use a chair/wedge); punching a bean bag; pull something heavy across the floor tied to a wheelchair; throw a large ball across the room.

Then sit in a circle, and take turns to demonstrate. Appoint one student to act as Penelope (or the person who will choose). When everyone has shown what they can do, he or she decides who is the king, and awards the gold crown. That person becomes Odysseus, and gets to choose the teams for the battle.

Introduction	We're going to see who is the STRONGest.
Purposes	*Assertiveness. Goal-directed behaviour. Choice-making.*

Variations

Have a genuine competition, with one kind of trial (but rig it so that different people win each week).

Visual impairment

Have a competition with audible or tactile consequences – e.g. pushing something heavy until it touches something that makes a sound. Alternatively, Penelope can stand on a chair with outstretched hands. Lift a heavy item until it touches her hands.

3. The Battle

Appoint one person (whoever has the crown, or who won the trial of strength) to be Odysseus. Another person is the leader of the rival team. Draw a line (or use a tape) down the middle of the room. Have everyone in a group, facing them with the line in between. They choose teams.

The teams must line up opposite one another, and have a 'fight'. You can use: water pistols; cushions thrown at each other; pushing one another into a corner; pushing wheelchairs against each other; act wrestling or boxing. Ring a bell when the fight is to start. Ring again for it to stop. Encourage students to fall down when 'hit'. Make sure there are lots of corpses.

Introduction	Now we KNOW who is the STRONGest. Now we KNOW who is the KING. But still there are enemies in our HOME. We'll have to FIGHT them, to make them GO away.
Purposes	*Interaction through contact. Choice-making. Goal-directed behaviour. Response to sound. Elicit feelings of anticipation, excitement, assertiveness. Experiencing and managing opposition / conflict.*

Variations

As an alternative to fighting, make some suitor figures for target practice (cardboard outlines of figures). Creep up on them and knock them down with water pistols/cushions/balls.

Visual impairment

Have a tactile 'battle strip' e.g. bubble wrap which people must push each other across. If you are using suitor figures, provide a sound dimension – e.g. make a 'revellers' tape' of people partying, drunken laughter, etc. It is switched off, and there is a scream/death gurgle every time a suitor is murdered.

4. Penelope

Each student must find a partner and greet them – e.g. slap or shake hands; reach out and touch; arm round shoulders. (Make sure that if you do the battle, you end with this). All join hands at the end.

Introduction	The FIGHT is FINISHED now. We've WON. LOOK for a FRIEND, and say hallo.
Purposes	*Bringing the group together. Interaction through reach and touch. Turn-taking – greeting. Goal-directed behaviour.*

5. Warp and Weft

This is a maypole type dance to represent Penelope's weaving. Pairs of students make the warp by standing in a line opposite each other, holding a strip. More mobile students and staff pass between them, alternately going under and over the strips, which are raised and lowered for them.

Introduction	Let's celebrate our homecoming with a DANCE.
Purposes	*Group awareness and interaction. Co-ordination and rhythm.*

Music suggestions	Dance music (folk, international or early music).
Slide suggestion	Pintoricchio: *Scenes from the Odyssey* (Penelope at her loom).
Resources	Long strips of coloured cloth, or crêpe paper.

With ITHACA, you have reached the end of the programme! You might want to celebrate with an all day party that recapitulates some of the activities – e.g. begin with Setting off; go into obstacle games, dances, massage, feasts.

Chapter 3

The Communication Framework

Odyssey Now is designed to encourage the active and intentional communication of feelings and ideas which grow out of interactions between people. Communication is a complex, many-layered process which is quite hard to analyse, especially when the people concerned lack the language skills to make their messages explicit, so we need to be very clear about the terms we use to describe it. What do we mean by *interaction, communication* and *intentionality*?

Interactions happen when people act together, either jointly, when everyone doing the same thing at the same time – or alternatively, when one person acts and another responds. The basis of an interaction is that one person becomes aware of another.

Communication happens when there is an exchange of information between people – where an idea, an intention, or a feeling is expressed by one person, and interpreted by another. A lot of what is communicated may not be deliberate – we constantly read meanings into the way people behave around us. However, for individuals to communicate effectively and independently, they must be capable of actively deciding to provide information to those they encounter. In other words, they must communicate *intentionally*. Many people with profound and multiple learning disabilities don't communicate with enough consistency and deliberation for us to be certain that they 'mean' us to understand particular messages. How does intentionality in communication develop, and how can we respond appropriately at each stage?

Communication Development

The model we are using as a basis for developing communication skills is based on work related to infant development, and identifies a continuum from behaviour which is pre-intentional, and non-symbolic, to behaviour which is deliberate, active and expressed through conventional symbolic forms such as words, signs or graphic symbols (Bates 1976; Coupe and Goldbart 1987; Dunst and Lowe 1986; Goldbart 1994; McLean and Snyder-McLean 1988).

PRE-INTENTIONAL		INTENTIONAL	
1. Reactive	2. Anticipatory	3. Intentional	4. Reciprocal

Figure 3.1 Stages of communication development

Level 1. At the first level, communication can be thought of as essentially *reactive* and *reflexive*. By changes in muscle tone, vocalising and facial expressions, a person communicates something about their state of being – hungry, tired, angry, excited, soothed. This behaviour is interpreted by the people around as if it 'meant' something. Meaning is therefore inferred rather than deliberately intended by the individual.

Level 2. The next stage is *anticipatory*. Gradually, the person learns to remember that one piece of behaviour is followed by a particular response, and begins to anticipate events – e.g. by fussing, reaching, smiling, holding arms up, withdrawing from a tickle. Intention and meaning/function is still inferred, rather than explicitly intended. The form of these signalling behaviours is often personal and idiosyncratic – familiar caregivers recognise the 'meaning', but an outside observer will not necessarily understand them (Campbell and Wilcox 1986; Rowland and Schweigert 1989). At Levels 1 and 2, communicative behaviour is 'concrete' and context-dependent, in that it is directly associated with events and activities, rather than standing for them as a true symbol does. For example, reaching towards a cup, whining and lip-smacking are behaviours whose forms express a state (thirst) directly. Once a person can say the word 'drink', on the other hand, they have acquired a conventional, abstract word that is understood by all English speakers. This is a true *symbol*, since there is no connection whatsoever between the form of the word, and the event it refers to. Behaviour at Levels 1 and 2 is described as *pre-intentional* and *pre-symbolic* – that is, the person is not yet deliberately and consciously trying to influence your response; and is not capable of expressing meanings through conventionalised words, signs, symbols or written text.

Our Role

With people functioning at Levels 1 and 2, our role is therefore to lead them to an understanding that they can affect others through the way they behave. We try to respond 'contingently' – i.e. immediately and appropriately, to the person's behaviour. By doing this repeatedly, the person comes to experience the consequences of his or her actions. We need to make opportunities and spaces in an interaction, to allow a person to produce consistent behaviour which can be 'shaped' through our consistent responses to it (Ware 1989; 1994).

Prompts, Cues and Imitation

At these stages, much behaviour may need to be *prompted* or *cued*. In a 'full' physical prompt, a person is moved through an action at the appropriate time. This can be faded gradually to a partial prompt, where the movement is started off for the person. At a later point still, only a cue may be needed – such as a touch on the arm. People functioning at Level 2 may be capable of *imitation*, where they are not directly prompted, but will copy a model of the behaviour.

Intensive Interactions

Prompted behaviours tend to be those which you introduce to the person with learning disabilities, because you have decided they are appropriate and functional. An alternative approach is to start from where the person is now, and try to enter their preoccupations, rather than introducing behaviour from outside (Nind and Hewett 1994; Sternberg and Owens 1985). If you are using intensive interaction, you will find a lot of similarity between the games described by Nind and Hewett and the activities in *Odyssey Now*, so that you could look at this project as a way of extending an individual's development by providing a narrative context in which the games take place. Other techniques involve moving with a person in close contact and following their rhythm, copying their movements at the same time, and copying them after a pause (Sternberg and Owens 1985).

Partners

Initially, people whose communication is primarily reactive are very dependent on the familiar people (usually adults) who take care of them. This does not, however, mean that they are unaware of their peers, or others with whom they come into contact. Even very passive communicators may show different behaviour with different people. Hence, right from the start, such individuals should be provided with opportunities to engage with all members of the social group to which they belong.

Intentional Interaction

Level 3. *Intentional* behaviour develops out of the second stage. The person begins to produce consistent behaviours with a clear expectation of a response from a communicative partner. Deciding if behaviour is intentional is still quite a subjective process – what looks like intent to one person may not do so to another. However, the presence of one or more of the following is generally taken as evidence (from Lock 1978):

- making eye contact – if someone looks at you either immediately before, during or immediately after vocalising, pointing, reaching or indicating something in the environment

- seeking proximity – if someone moves closer to you before he or she acts

- alteration of behaviour in response to a partner's behaviour – e.g. if someone tries whining, *then* reaching to get attention, when the partner fails to respond

- ritualisation of behaviour – a reach changes from the full arm, to extension from the elbow; fussing noises become shorter and more regular, taking on the characteristics of a definite sound which functions as a protest (Bates, Benigni, Bretherton, Camaioni and Volterra 1979).

The difference between this stage, and the preceding one, as the difference between reaching as an end in itself, where a child's attention is directed towards the object she wants, the reach is fully extended, she leans forward, vocalising; and reaching which acts as a signal. In this case, the child leans back in her chair, extends her arm from the elbow towards the cup, but looks at the adult. She may also alternate gaze and/or reach between the cup and the adult.

Intentional communication may be regarded as a particular type of purposeful, *goal-directed* behaviour, where a person is clearly using behaviour as a means to an end.

Level 4. Once a person has reached the stage of producing intentional behaviour, they have grasped the fact that they can make things happen through communication, and that other people can respond to them. However, they may not yet understand that communication is *reciprocal* – it is about sharing experiences, and empathising with others, to the extent that we learn to read how others are thinking and feeling, and to adapt our behaviour accordingly. Entering into reciprocity with another person enables fluent, relevant communication, which involves a great deal of inference and prediction (Sperber and Wilson 1986). Once someone has attained this level, they can start to use words, signs, pictures or symbols to communicate about events removed from the immediate context, to describe thoughts and feelings, and to handle more abstract ideas.

At Levels 3 and 4, the way people communicate becomes more conventional and recognisable – points, waves, extending objects in exchanges, some 'natural' gestures that represent events and actions, such as clapping to request a particular song. People may also start to develop a small vocabulary of words, signs, or symbols – usually associated with particular ongoing events. Gradually these come to acquire full symbolic status, used to denote a class of objects (e.g. *dogs* – rather than one particular dog) and to refer to absent objects and people.

Our Role

Once we are confident that a certain behaviour is intentionally produced, we can begin to encourage more conventional, less idiosyncratic forms, for example by prompting and cueing people to produce a fully extended arm reach, rather than a partial extension; (e.g. modelling a sign for DRINK). At this point, it becomes appropriate for caregivers and partners to withdraw a little, and provide the spaces and the challenges to enable people to become more independent as communicators. Rather than always responding immediately (as is appropriate at earlier levels), we may introduce some uncertainty and change into the situation, so that individuals are not so dependent on predictable routines. Too much need-fulfilment at this stage can lead to passive dependence on others, just as failure to respond will do at Levels 1 and 2. This process, of providing the right level of support for development to take place, and then gradually withdrawing it as people become competent, has been described as *scaffolding* (Bruner 1983).

Prompting, Cueing and Imitation

People do not acquire intentional behaviour right across the board, in all communication contexts. Once a behaviour is used intentionally, it is likely to occur spontaneously – that is, the person initiates it him or herself, in the appropriate situation, without needing to be prompted. When acquiring new behaviours, however, a person may need some help to integrate them into their existing repertoire.

This model of development is progressive and hierarchical; it is like starting with the foundations of a block of flats, and building upwards. However, there is another way of thinking about development and that is by broadening the range of someone's experience – like an extension which adds rooms on the same floor.

We need to think simultaneously about raising the levels of intention and spontaneity, and broadening the *forms* of behaviours that people can use as communicative signals and the range of *meanings* they can signal, and the *contexts* (people and situations) within which they interact. One way of doing this is to identify a number of different questions that you can ask about a person's communication skills – the **if** question, the **how** question, the **what** question, the **who** question, the **when** question and the question of **our response**.

Whenever we are in contact with another person, we have to make a set of decisions which correspond to these questions, and our answers allow us to make judgements about the level of intentionality, form, meaning and context of their communication. So we have to think about **if** someone is trying to communicate *(intentionality)*; **how** they are doing it *(form)* **what** someone wants to tell us *(meaning)*; **who** they are communicating with; what **our response** should be *(our role)*, and **when** they are choosing, or not choosing to communicate *(context)*. It may look very complicated, but actually it is no more than we are all doing intuitively when we meet different people, in different situations, and adapt our communication styles accordingly.

We have already analysed the development of intentionality, and our role in facilitating communication. Figures 3.2 and 3.3 illustrate the forms and meanings of communication which are available to people before they develop any form of spoken, signed, or written language.

How People Communicate – Forms

People can communicate effectively in all sorts of different ways. If we can become aware of the channels of communication that individuals are using, we may be able to increase our own ability to respond to them, and then gradually establish systematic 'habits' of communication which can function as recognisable signals.

Figure 3.2 provides some examples of the range of communicative behaviour at different stages of development. It is important to remember that, once we develop language, and come to depend primarily on one type of communication (say, speech or sign language), we do not stop communicating in other ways, such as facial expressions, gestures and sounds.

What People Communicate – Meanings and Purposes

Elizabeth Bates (1976), in her study of infants' communicative behaviours, noticed that most could be categorised into two functions, or purposes: either asking for things or telling you what to do *(Requests/commands)*, or drawing your attention to something *(Comments)*. Requests and commands are alike in that they express what

PRE-INTENTIONAL STAGE

These communicative behaviours are used in the pre-intentional stage, and they continue to be significant once communication is intentional, and when language has developed.

Body attitude	e.g. Arousal, habituation, relaxation. Approach and withdrawal. Aggression.
Using hands	e.g. Touching. Reaching. Pulling. Use of another person – e.g. moving someone's hand to open a door.
Facial expressions	
Eye gaze	
Vocalisation	
Using objects	e.g. Banging, throwing, giving.

INTENTIONAL STAGE

These behaviours are normally associated with intentional communication.

Gestures	e.g. Waving goodbye, hand-to-mouth 'oh dear'.
Pointing	To objects, places, and people.
Use of pictures	e.g. Bringing a picture of the TV to show she wants it turned on.
Speech	Recognisable words.
Sign	Manual signs from a sign language.

Figure 3.2. How people communicate

SELF-RELATED		OTHER-RELATED
Requests	**Negation**	**Comments**
for Person	Protest	re a Person
for Object	Refuse	re an Object
	Deny	re an Action
for Action (command)		re an Event
for Attention		
for Assistance		
for Interaction	Non-Existence	re Non-existence
(contact, play,		re Errors and
conversation)	Errors and	Mistakes
	Mistakes	
		Name
Question		People
(ask for information,		Objects
permission, answers)		Places
		Events
Express States		
and Feelings		**Turn-taking**
Pleasure		Offer objects
Humour		Take objects
Affection		
Excitement		Social routines
		(greeting and farewell)
Grief		
Pain		Games
Anger		
Fear		
Confusion		Initiate
Boredom		Answer
Frustration		(Yes/No signals)

Figure 3.3. What people communicate

the child wants – they are self-related. Comments, on the other hand, reflect children's interest in and engagement with the world around them. At the earliest stage, these behaviours do not involve words or signs, but pre-linguistic behaviours such as vocalisations, points and reaches. At a slightly later stage, when children start to develop language, they begin to use words or signs, not only to draw attention to objects and people, but to give them names. Naming, according to this model, grows out of the earlier function which we have chosen to call Commenting.

Figure 3.3 lists the functions, or meanings, which have been identified in both the pre-linguistic stage and early language (Sternberg, Ehrens, Leferts and Eloranta 1988). There are five main categories: **Requests, Comments, Feelings, Turn-Taking** and **Negation.**

Requests include *commands*, which are essentially requests for actions, interactions, or attention. (i.e. the child is wanting you to do something, rather than wanting an object) and *questions*, which emerge relatively late in development and are usually regarded as specialised requests – for information. *Choice-making* can be included under the heading of Requests: where someone is provided with alternatives to reach towards, name, or look at, for example.

Comments are defined as any attempt to draw your attention to something with an existence outside the person: an event, an object, a person, or the fact that something is not there. Comments may also draw attention to mistakes (such as putting a coat on the wrong peg) – these are an important source of jokes and humour. Once a vocabulary (of signs, words, or symbols) is acquired, a person can *name* people, events and objects.

Expression of Feelings is a self-related category, which may or may not involve intentional communication. People show how they feel by their posture, facial expression and vocalisations – they may also be able to sign OK, HAPPY, ANGRY.

Turn-Taking is engaged in for its own sake. Like comments, turn-taking behaviours necessarily involve awareness of something, or someone, other than the self. People may develop consistent behaviours associated with giving and taking of objects, such as extending a hand, and vocalising. These activities are parallel to conversations, which can occur pre-verbally, when people make sounds to one another – or, if they are deaf or totally non-vocal, exchange gestures, facial expressions or signs. Well-known turn-taking games include peek-a-boo, or handclapping. Under the heading of Turn-Taking we include yes–no responses. These will not be produced by people who are at a pre-intentional stage, but are very important signals to develop for making choices, and indicating consent.

Negation This fifth 'meaning' in fact relates to the four other functions: Requests, Comments, Turn-taking and Feelings. Rejections, protests and refusals express something the child does *not* want, or a command *not* to do something. Indicating that something is not there, or is wrong is a negative sort of comment. Shaking the head, saying no, or averting gaze when asked questions that demand yes–no responses, is participating in turn-taking. And, of course, negations are often associated with the expression of feelings. Negation is included as a separate category because it is so important in developing a sense of identity, in making choices, and in becoming independent.

Using the Communication Framework

All the games in *Odyssey Now* have specified purposes, which link back to this framework. They attempt to develop intentional and goal-directed behaviour, elicit contrasting moods and feelings, implicate one or more communicative functions, and demand the use of a range of communicative modalities. We hope that by playing these games, you will be providing an appropriate context for the use of these skills. However, hope is an inadequate basis for effective practice with students who have profound and multiple learning disabilities! In the section on record-keeping (Chapter 5), we have suggested a way in which you could use the framework to set objectives for individuals, and to monitor what happens in the sessions.

Chapter 4

Multi-Sensory Presentations

Foregrounds and Backgrounds

In *Odyssey Now* we have tried to make use of visual, auditory and tactile stimuli, to create atmospheres that are richly evocative, and to ensure that people can benefit from all of the sensory channels that are available to them. The basic techniques and philosophy of multi-sensory presentations are described in *Communication as Curriculum* (Park, Robinson and Williams 1989). What we have taken from this programme is the idea of using discrete types of music, visual art and smell as cues for particular events: the episodes form the story. We have also applied the principle of *foregrounding.* which was developed by Park (1991; 1992) in the context of a communication course run for adults with profound and multiple learning disabilities. In the weekly sessions, it was noticed that the visual contrast of a symbol card in torchlight against a black background seemed to have a visual attraction for the students. Towards the end of the first term, it became apparent that these foreground/background contrasts might also be developed through sound, touch, movement and smell. By these means, a 'sensory matrix' might be devised to assist staff in developing more effectively stimulating environments. Furthermore, this strategy might be easily transferable to the students' home environments, and allow residential care workers and others to make suggestions and contribute ideas about the lives of the people in their care.

It should be added that there was no interest in developing a 'stimulus free' environment to minimise 'distraction' – if anything, the aim was the reverse, namely to systematically enrich the environment. Nor did the contrasts need to be strongly discriminated. For example, since background noise of some sort is inevitable, was it possible – or appropriate – to 'overlay' the background noise with a particular type of music? Is it relevant that a classroom may have a faint but recognisable odour? Was it possible – or appropriate – to have a background scent? It was felt that these issues were worth exploring, since none of the students had any independent mobility and were totally dependent upon others for care routines and leisure activities and for the range of their sensory experiences.

Figure 4.1 provides a schematic outline of multisensory input in one of the episodes from the project ('Nausicaa').

Vision

During the communication course described above, careful attention was paid to the optimal presentations for eliciting visual attention and visual tracking. This was because although the students could all *see*, none of them seemed to be able to *look*. In this context, symbol cards were designed with fluorescent borders (foreground) and presented against a black background, to enhance the contrast. In 'Nausicaa', one aspect of each activity is visually foregrounded for students: first the painting, against the background of a darkened room; then the 'rocks' (wedge construction) against which they will crash; then the various foods in the second activity; and finally the picture again.

Hearing

Just as the students appeared to be able to *see* but not to *look*, they seemed to be able to *hear* without being able to *listen* (each student's hearing status had been confirmed). Again, the problem was considered in terms of enabling the student to distinguish between foreground sound (the teacher's voice, for example) and background sound – people coming and going, doors slamming. One way of providing consistent background sound was through carefully selected music (with the caveat that too often, individuals who live in institutions may have become desensitised to the 'auditory background' of a TV or radio which is left on continuously). In 'Nausicaa', auditory foregrounds are provided by the specific spoken introductions to each activity. Auditory backgrounds consist of the music accompanying the picture and sounds and vocalisations made by others.

	Vision	Hearing	Touch	Smell
Introduction				
Foreground	picture	'look'	–	–
Background	darkroom	music	seating position	seaweed
Setting Off				
Foreground	picture	'we're going in a boat'	movement to and – fro	
Background	dark room	everyday sounds	seating position	incense
Storm				
Foreground	'rocks'	storm noises	'rain'	–
Background	blue light	everyday involuntary sounds	seating position	incense
Banquet				
Foreground	food items	food names	eating	food scents
Background	yellow light or picture	music	seating position	incense
Winding Down				
Foreground	picture	'look'	–	–
Background	dark room	music	seating position	incense

Figure 4.1 Sensory matrix – 'Nausicaa' episode

Touch

The students' foreground for the sense of touch was massage of hands, head, or feet, set against the 'background' tactile kinaesthetic experience of their own body position. Seen from this perspective, it was clear that students were spending a disproportionate amount of time in the same position in wheelchairs. With advice from a physiotherapist, it was possible to devise a number of alternative positions for each individual for the various activities, for example, supine for hand massage, supported sitting for morning tea. In the *Odyssey Now* activities, it may be too difficult to change seating positions regularly for individuals, but there are a number of occasions where physical contact is foregrounded in games.

Smell

Foregrounds and backgrounds here referred to those scents which were close up – the massage oils, scent of a member of staff, etc. – and those general pervasive odours (which in this case was the faint but noticeable one of a damp carpet!). In *Odyssey Now*, you can use a different background scent for each episode with incense sticks, massage oils, strong-smelling plants, food, and other stimuli such as earth and seaweed.

Using the Multi-Sensory Framework

By ensuring that the project provides a range of sensory experiences, we are trying to do two things. One is to create a particular atmosphere for each episode of the story. We hope that people who may not be able to follow a narrative can learn to recognise and respond to a series of contrasting events. The second aim is to cater for the needs of individuals. The games, the music, the pictures and scents intrinsically stimulate vision, hearing, touch and smell, so that everyone should be able to build up some contrastive sensory associations to the episodes. It is important to ensure that opportunities are consistently provided for people to actively participate, using appropriate modalities of communication. For this reason, we suggest that consideration of sensory preferences should form part of the process of setting objectives for individuals, as described in the following chapter on record-keeping.

Chapter 5

Record-Keeping

Odyssey Now can simply be a leisure activity for fun. However, if the programme is to be used as a way of developing communication skills, it is important to choose activities that are relevant to individuals, and to keep some kind of record of responses.

You may already have a system of goal-setting and record-keeping which can be used in association with the programme. Feel free to adapt our suggestions to your own situation.

Organising the Programme

Planning Meeting

Before you run the programme, you will need one or two planning meetings with staff in which you can:

- choose the episodes

- discuss resources

- set individual goals

- decide what tasks staff will undertake in each session (room management). It's a good idea to rotate these. For each session you need to decide who will *set it up*; who will *run the session*; who will *act as record-keeper*. If you are very short of staff, record keeping can be carried out at transition points between activities.

Try to allow yourselves plenty of time at this stage for sharing ideas, and really focusing on individual needs.

Run-Throughs

Before you finally decide on running the programme on a long-term basis, try out the episodes you have chosen once or twice. If they don't seem to work as you had hoped, you may want to change them. Bear in mind, however, that people with severe disabilities may need to have time to acclimatise to new situations and challenges before they will be able to respond really positively.

Use these sessions to obtain baselines for individual goals.

Reviewing How it Went

If you can organise time for a separate review meeting, do it! If this isn't possible, use the 'Winding Down' period of the session, while people are looking at the slide, listening to music and relaxing. Talk quietly about the session, make notes on what happened, and look quickly at the group record sheet to determine any 'next steps' for the group or individuals. You could also single out one or two individuals each session, and use the 'Winding Down' period to sit with them and review together what they did.

Decision-making: Matching Activities and Individual Needs

This is a process of setting objectives for individuals for each session, taking into account their level of communication, and their sensory preferences. The record form for individuals – Form 2 (see Appendix 2) – specifies existing achievements, communication objectives, the behaviours you plan to encourage during the programme, and staff roles. The following procedures can be used as a guide to completing the form.

For those who like tick charts, this is an alternative to the descriptive format. You could use both! Under Meanings, note down what you think the person is communicating (you could use the list in Figure 3.3 as a guide). Tick the boxes to indicate the range of behaviours that he person is using.

Before You Start

Step 1. Starting points: The What and How of Communication

Think about *what* meanings each person in the group currently seems to be communicating, and *how* he or she is communicating that meaning. Think about sensory preferences, and how foregrounds and backgrounds can be used. Use Figures 3.3 and 4.1 as a guide.

Are any of these meanings communicated *intentionally*, i.e. consistently, and with an apparent awareness of other people? For example, making eye contact with you; moving nearer to you; always using a particular behaviour in a particular context. Use the levels suggested to provide an indication.

This work could be done before the planning meeting. Ask the staff involved to jot down their impressions, and consult with speech therapists/physiotherapists.

At The Planning Meeting

Step 2. Where next?

What do you think would be an appropriate development for the person?

This could be to extend the range of how and what they communicate: by encouraging them to use their hands or voice or body contact; or encouraging them to develop a 'meaning' that they do not seem to be using, e.g. a way of saying no, a way of asking for attention; or by encouraging them to use the skills they have with a different person – a friend rather than the usual member of staff, for example.

Or you may want to try to develop the level of intentionality (Levels 3 and 4) by encouraging any spontaneous attempts to reach, touch, push away, and prompting them to make eye contact.

Think of one or two goals which could potentially be developed through the programme.

At the Planning Meeting (continued)

Step 3. Which games?

Look at the episodes you are planning to use from *Odyssey Now*.

What do you think are the most relevant activities for the person? How might a game be adapted for someone's particular needs? Which elements of the sensory presentation would you expect to be most important for that person?

For each session, choose 1 game per person which you think could be used to develop an appropriate communication skill. Make sure that you spread record keeping so that you are observing at least one person per game, and that every group member is observed at least once.

Step 4. What to look for

Decide what *kind* of communication behaviour you will aim to elicit from the person in response to the game, and how you will elicit it (e.g. through prompting, modelling, waiting). You may want to revise this once you have done some initial observations (base line); you may decide to delay decisions until after you have done so. This step is included here because it is often difficult to gather staff together for more than one thorough planning meeting.

Repeat this procedure for each person in the group for whom it is relevant. Enter the findings and decisions on the individual record form.

At the First Run-Through

Step 5. First impressions

The first run-through of the session is an opportunity to obtain a record of how people respond to the activities you have chosen, *without your intervention*. Use the group record form to describe briefly what each person did in response to the game.

Use the review period (after the session, or during 'Winding Down' activity) to revise any goals for individuals which look to be inappropriate.

From Then On

People often don't do what we expect or predict, and sometimes their spontaneous behaviour surprises us. Be prepared to change your goals in response to any new behaviour which looks as though it is advancing someone's communication skills – in whatever direction.

Step 7. What's happening this time?

Use the group record form (Form 3, see Appendix 2) to describe briefly what each person did in response to the game.

Step 8. Next steps

Use the review period (after the session, or during 'Winding Down' activity) to discuss what people noticed, and to revise any goals for individuals which are now inappropriate, need modifying, or have been achieved.

Keeping a Record During Sessions

The aim of record-keeping is *not* to provide a complete breakdown of what each person is doing throughout the session. We advocate a selective approach, which allows you to focus on particular individuals only during particular games.

Form 3 (Appendix 2) is an example of a group record, which can be used to note down observations made during or after the session.

Chapter 6

Odyssey Now and the National Curriculum[1]

Using *Odyssey Now* as a framework, the teacher of pupils with severe and profound and multiple disabilities will have the opportunity to make reference to most of the 11 subject areas of the National Curriculum.

The National Curriculum references included in this section are all from the January 1995 edition of the Department for Education *Key Stages 1 and 2 of the National Curriculum*: these are in effect from August 1995. Each of the eleven subjects is prefaced by a 'Common Requirements' section: this introduction explains that 'the statement on access in the section on Common Requirements increases the scope for teachers to provide such pupils [i.e. those with special educational needs] with appropriately challenging work at each "key stage."'.

The statement on access reads:

> For the small number of pupils who may need the provision, material may be selected from earlier or later key stages where this is necessary to enable pupils to progress and demonstrate achievement. Such material should be presented in contexts suitable to the pupil's age.

In the light of this statement, and because most of the people who have been using this material work with children with severe and profound learning disabilities, all of the selected references (with the exception of references to Modern Foreign Language (Key Stage 3), History (Key Stage 2), and Swimming (Physical Education, Key Stage 2)) are to Key Stage 1. Subject areas are listed alphabetically.

Under each subject area, examples are given of activities from episode one – 'Cyclops' – of *Odyssey Now*. There will, of course, be

---

1   Material from the National Curriculum is Crown copyright and is reproduced by permission of the Controller of HMSO.

many other ways of making reference to the National Curriculum areas using this material, and the activities listed below are only those which have already been tried, or are already in practice.

Art

Investigating and Making

2. In order to develop visual perception, pupils should be taught the creative, imaginative and practical skills needed to:

    (a) express ideas and feelings

    (b) record observations

    (c) design and make images and artefacts.

    Examples: make a mask from the 'Cyclops' to wear in the 'One Eye' game; make a giant 'Cyclops' figure from papier mache; make a mixed-media collage of the 'boulder escape' scene.

3. In order to develop visual literacy, pupils should be taught about the different ways in which ideas, feelings, and meanings are communicated in visual form.

    Example: show the slide *Ulysses Deriding Polyphemus* and choose some music to go with it, for example the theme tune of the film *Jaws*. If you do not have the slide, get a poster of a giant – or make one. Experiment with ways of creating different moods by using pictures and music (and scent, of course).

Design and Technology

1. Pupils should be given opportunities to develop their design and technology capability through:

    (a) assignments in which they design and make products

    (b) focused practical tasks in which they develop and practise particular skills and knowledge.

    Example: make a many-textured blanket (i.e. a blanket made of squares of contrasting materials such as corduroy, imitation fur, sheepskin etc.) that can be used in the 'Sheep Escape' game, and could also be used for classroom sensory activities.

English

Speaking and Listening

1(a) Pupils should be given opportunities to talk for a range of purposes, including: imaginative play and drama, reading and listening to nursery rhymes and poetry.

Example: all the activities of *Odyssey Now* come under this heading.

Reading

1(d) The literature read should cover the following categories:

- poems and stories with familiar settings and those based upon imaginary or fantasy worlds

- retelling of traditional folk and fairy stories

- stories and poems from a range of cultures

- stories and poems that are particularly challenging in terms of length or vocabulary.

2(c) In understanding and responding to stories and poems, pupils should be given opportunities to:

- hear stories and poems read aloud frequently and regularly, including some longer, more challenging material.

Each episode has a storyline which can be retold everytime the episode is used.

Writing

1(b) Pupils should be given opportunities to write in response to a variety of stimuli, including stories, poems, classroom experiences and personal experience.

Example: make a rebus or pictographic story book of the activity sequence of the 'Cyclops' episode, showing pupils participating in the activities; make symbol cards for Odysseus and the Cyclops. Use the letters from 'Odysseus', 'Cyclops' and/or the real names of the group as a basis for artwork.

Geography

1. Pupils should be given opportunities to:

    (c) become aware that the world extends beyond their own locality, both within and outside the United Kingdom, and that the places they study exist within this border geographical context, e.g. within a town, a region, a country.

Example: collect pictures and photographs of Greece – ancient and modern – and use it as a start for a project on Greek culture: its food, music, dances, ways of life, etc.

History

There are three 'Areas of Study' and five 'Key Elements', and it is stated that these should be taught together. The following are examples:

Areas of Study

2. Pupils should be taught about the lives of different kinds of famous men and women, including personalities drawn from British history, e.g. rulers, saints, artists, engineers, explorers, inventors, pioneers.

Key Elements

2. Range and depth of historical knowledge and understanding.

    (a) pupils should be taught about aspects of the past through stories from different periods and cultures, including stories and eyewitness accounts of historical events.

4. Historical enquiry:

    (a) how to find out about aspects of the past from a range of sources of information, including artefacts, pictures and photographs, adults talking about their own pets, written sources, and buildings and sites.

Example: as described in the Geography example.

Key Stage 2, Study Unit 4

The way of life, beliefs and achievements of the ancient Greeks, and the legacy of ancient Greek civilization to the modern world.

Example: we would suggest that the use of *Odyssey Now* illustrates this!

Information Technology

1. Pupils should be given opportunities to:

   (a) use a variety of IT equipment and software, including microcomputers and various keyboards, to carry out a variety of functions in a range of contexts.

3. Controlling and modelling:

   (c) use IT-based models or simulations to explore aspects of real and imaginary situations.

Mathematics

Shape, Space and Measures

1. Pupils should be given opportunities to:

   (a) gain a wide range of practical experience using a variety of materials

   (b) use IT devices, e.g. programmable toys, turtle graphics packages

2. Understanding and using patterns and properties of shape:

   (b) make common 3-D and 2-D shapes and models, working with increasing care and accuracy; begin to classify shapes according to mathematical criteria.

Example: make 2-D and 3-D boats for a mixed-media collage of a sea picture.

Modern Foreign Languages: Key Stage 3

Part One: Learning And Using The Target Language

1. Communicating in the target language.

4. Cultural awareness – pupils should be given opportunities to:

    (a) work with authentic materials, including newspapers, magazines, books, films, radio and television, from the countries of communities of the target language.

Example: one staff member brought some slides of Greek coastline and these were used, with Greek music, to create a different atmosphere in the classroom. It is the perfect setting to eat baklava!

Music

1. Pupils should be given opportunities to:

    (a) use sounds and respond to music individually, in pairs, in groups and as a class

    (b) make appropriate use of IT to record sounds.

Example: make a video of the group listening to the music in the 'Setting Off' and 'Winding Down' activities; make an audiotape of everyone singing along with Rod Stewart's 'Sailing'!

3. The repertoire chosen for performing and listening should extend pupils' musical experience and knowledge, and develop their appreciation of the richness of our diverse cultural heritage. It should include music in a variety of ways:

    (a) from different times and cultures

    (b) by well known composers and performers, past and present.

Examples: the music suggestions for the Cyclops episode are deliberately varied: Mussorgsky, Liszt, Orff, film scores with chase music such as *Jaws*. Encourage staff and, if possible, pupils to make other suggestions: Greek music such as the soundtrack from *Zorba the Greek*, for example.

Performing and Composing

> 5(e) Pupils should be taught to improvise musical patterns, e.g. to invent and change patterns whilst playing and singing.

> 5(g) Pupils should be taught to use sounds to create musical effects, e.g. to suggest a machine or a walk through a forest.

Example: experiment with making variations on the 'Setting Off' activity by creating the effects of a sea voyage: switch on a fan, use a parachute or space blanket to make waves, sway from side to side, spray people – gently! – with water from a plant sprayer, and have a soundtrack of waves breaking on the shore as a background!

Listening and Appraising

Pupils should be taught how to:

(a) recognise how sounds can be made in different ways, e.g. by blowing, plucking, shaking, vocalising

(c) recognise that music comes from different times and places

(d) respond to musical elements, and the changing character and mood of a piece of music by means of dance or other suitable forms of expression.

Example: use the 'Setting Off' activity to make a song or chant about being on a boat, going home, etc. Use drums and tambourines, and make a recording of it.

Physical Education

Games

Pupils should be taught:

(a) simple competitive games, including how to play them as individuals and, when ready, in pairs and in small groups

(b) to develop and practise a variety of ways of sending (including throwing, striking, rolling and bouncing) receiving and travelling with a ball and other similar games equipment

(c) elements of games that include running, chasing, dodging, avoiding, and awareness of space and other players.

Example: play the 'Boulder Escape' game and invent variations of it.

Gymnastic Activities

Pupils should be taught:

(a) different ways of performing the basic actions of travelling using hands and feet, turning, rolling, jumping, balancing, swinging and climbing, both on the floor and using apparatus

(b) to link a series of actions both on the floor and using apparatus, and how to repeat them.

Example: in the 'Sheep Escape' game, explore how may ways in which it is possible to move out of the 'cave', avoiding the blinded Cyclops: rolling, crawling, on the back, side, front, etc.

Dance

Pupils should be taught:

(a) to perform control, co-ordination, balance, poise and elevation in the basic actions of travelling, jumping, turning, gesture and stillness

(b) to perform movements or patterns, including some form existing dance traditions

(c) to explore moods and feelings and to develop their response to music through dances, by using rhythmic responses and contrasts of speed, shape, direction and level.

Example: use the game of 'Grandmother's Footsteps' (a 'Moving On' activity suggestion) to develop variety of movement. Invent a 'Cyclops' dance, where everyone stands in a circle and the person who is 'it' weaves in and out, finally touching someone who then takes over. Use the music from the film *Zorba the Greek* and design a dance for it.

Swimming: Key Stage 2

Pupils should be taught:

(b) to develop confidence in the water, and how to rest, float and adopt support positions.

Example: one school has used the 'Sirens' episode successfully in the hydrotherapy pool, using all of the activities as 'swimming games'. This can also be done with the 'Cyclops' episode, where, for example, pupils and staff have to get from one end of the pool to the other without being touched or splashed by the 'Cyclops' ('Boulder Escape'). The 'One Eye' game can be played with an inflatable toy as the 'Eye'.

Science

Experimental and Investigative Science

2. Obtaining evidence – pupils should be taught:

(a) to explore using appropriate senses.

Example: in the 'Sheep Escape' game, make the room dark, and fill it with wedges, mats, and large plastic balls. How does a familiar environment change in the dark, and when filled with different things?

Materials and their Properties

1. Grouping materials – pupils should be taught:

(a) to use their senses to explore and recognise the similarities and differences between materials.

Example: having made a many-textured blanket for the 'Sheep Escape' game, make a number of similar blankets, either of one, two or more textures. These can be used on the floor, for laying or walking on, or as a wallcovering or arras, and attached to the classroom wall. Pupils can be encouraged to compare the textures.

Appendix I

Using Poetry with Odyssey Now

'All the past – history, myth, and legend – exists everywhere and for all of us: we are in it, and it is in us.' (W.J. Smith, from the Introduction to *Moral Tales* by Jules Laforgue)

It is generally accepted that Homer lived somewhere between 760 and 650 BC. This would make his *Odyssey* over 2500 years old. It is supposed that Homer was the first person to create a written version of the oral account which may have existed for many years before that. The identity of Homer the poet, however, remains shrouded in mystery. Rubens and Taplin (1989) discuss and reject a long-standing theory of multiple authorship of the Odyssey in favour of 'a single maker' (Rubens and Taplin, 1989, p.27). The poet and scholar Robert Graves suggests that 'the light, humorous, naive, spirited touch of the Odyssey is almost certainly a woman's' (Graves, 1985, p.365), and remarks that the portrayal of the character Nausicaa may even be an autobiographical sketch. This uncertainty of identity once led the writer George Bernard Shaw to quip that the Odyssey had not been written by Homer, but by someone else with the same name.

However, after Homer whoever, he, she, or they may be – from Euripedes, who wrote his verse play *Cyclops* in the fourth century BC, to Derek Walcott, whose play *The Odyssey* was published in 1993 – there is a line of writers and artists who have constantly re-told, adapted, and alluded to characters and episodes in the *Odyssey*. For example, the figure of Odysseus appears in the poetry of Ovid (first century AD), of Spenser (sixteenth century), to Ezra Pound and W.H. Auden in the twentieth century. As 'Ulysses', Odysseus even makes an appearance in Canto 26 of Dante's *Inferno* (early fourteenth century), in the eighth Circle of Hell, eternally wrapped in flames as a punishment 'for the ambush of the horse' or the deception of the Trojan Horse. Rubens and Taplin (1989), in their book *An Odyssey Round Odysseus*, discuss this process of perpetual re-invention, and say of these subsequent works: 'they are like the fruiting of a very ancient tree: the trunk remains, the olives are new every year'.

The poems in this reference list are some of those 'olives'. It also contains a few references that are concerned with sea travel (for example the Old English poems 'The Seafarer' and 'The Wayfarer') that are not actually derived from or inspired by the *Odyssey*, but are evocative of one or more aspects of it. The poetry has been used in two main ways:

1. As part of a 'Setting Off' or 'Winding Down' session, it can be read with accompanying music and/or colour slide. For example, e.e.

cummings' 'poem 9' – which is only four lines long – can be read, and signed while showing a slide such as *Sunrise with Seamonsters* and the music of Vaughan Williams' *Lark Ascending*. Add an incense stick and it can be very evocative. Participants can be encouraged to learn part or all of the poem in words or signs, or both.

2. As part of an activity; for example, in the 'Sirens' episode, when someone is being wrapped up in a parachute in the 'Charybdis' game, the others can chant one or two lines from Spenser's *Faerie Queene* that actually describes Charybdis: 'That is the Gulfe of Greedinesse, they say', and so on. Spenser's sixteenth century English may look and sound a little strange, but using the music of the words can contribute greatly to the atmosphere and the fun of the game.

Most of the references are generally available, and all of the poetry can be found at The Poetry Library (Royal Festival Hall, South Bank Centre, London SE1 8XX. Tel: 0171-921-0943). Membership of the poetry library is free.

Poetry References

Arnold, Matthew
The *Collected Poems* (Oxford: Oxford University Press, 1982) includes the sonnet sequence 'To Marguerite', which uses imagery of the sea.

Auden, W.H.
The poem 'Circe' (*Collected Poems*, London: Faber and Faber, 1985) is a description of Circe's island. Parts of it have been recited at the beginning of the 'Circe' episode, to the accompaniment of slow and languid music ('Wish You Were Here' by Pink Floyd), and showing Botticelli's picture *Venus and Mars*.

Borges, Jorge Luis
The poem 'Ars Poetica' refers to Ulysses and Ithaca, and is in Borges' *Selected Poems 1923–1967* (trans and ed by N.T. Digiovanni. London: Allen Lane, 1972).

Bunting, Basil
Collected Poems (Moyer Bell, 1985). Bunting's poems contain several striking references to the sea.

Cavafy, C.P.
Collected Poems (London: Chatto and Windus 1990) contains the poem 'Ithaka' (trans. E. Keeley and P. Sherrard).

Crossley-Holland, K. (ed)
The *Oxford Book of Travel Verse* (Oxford: Oxford University Press, 1989) contains many poems of sea journeys. It also contains Laurie Lee's poem 'Home From Abroad' which can be used in the 'Ithaca' section.

cummings, e.e.
'poem 9' (1964) from the volume *73 poems* (London: Faber and Faber, 1985) has been used as described on page 86.

Day Lewis, Cecil
'Selected Poems' (London: Penguin 1974) contains the poem 'Nearing again the legendary isle', an ironic poem about the sirens, grown old and toothless.

Donne, John
'A Storm at Sea' can be found in *Collected Poems* (Oxford: Oxford University Press, 1992) and is a wry description of a storm at sea and its effect on the behaviour of the passengers.

du Bellay, Joachim
'The Regrets', a poem about homecoming, uses the imagery of Ulysses, and can be found in a volume of the same name (*The Regrets*, translated by C.H. Sisson, London: Carcanet Press, 1984)

Durrell, Lawrence
His poem 'On Ithaca Standing' can be found in his *Collected Poems 1931–1974*, (London: Faber and Faber, 1980).

Euripides
The verse play *Cyclops*, written sometime in the fourth century BC, is based upon the Cyclops episode of the Odyssey, and is a rich resource for the 'Cyclops' episode.

Ewart, Gavin
His poem 'Circe' is in *The Faber Book of Blue Verse* (ed Gavin Ewart. London: Faber and Faber, 1990). Please be aware, if you are taking this book into school, that it is a book of blue verse!

Flecker, J.E.
'The Old Ships' pp.253–4 *Come Hither*, vol.11. A collection of rhymes and poems (ed. W de le Mare 1957) (London: Kestrel Books).

Hamer, Richard (ed)
A Choice of Anglo-Saxon Verse (London: Faber and Faber, 1970) contains a verse translation of 'The Seafarer' and 'The Wanderer.' These are very evocative poems about journeys: the book has parallel text for anyone wanting to recite them in Old English!

Hopkins, Gerald Manley
'The Wreck of the Deutschland' is a long poem about a shipwreck (*Collected Poems*, London: Penguin, 1981). Sections of it have been used in the 'Sirens' episode, accompanied by sound effects of the sea and the *Shipwreck* picture by Turner.

Horace
In Horace's *Collected Odes* (London: Penguin, 1990), Epode XVII contains descriptions of Odysseus (called 'Ulysses' by Horace) on the island of Circe. The Odes were written in the first century BC.

Jones, Selwyn Russell
Jones's title poem 'Driftwood Odyssey' (Winchester: Sarsen Press 1990) uses the imagery of the odyssey of human life.

MacNiece, Louis
His *Collected Poems* (London: Faber and Faber, 1979) contains 'Day of Returning', describing Odysseus' feelings for his own country. The final poem, 'Thalassa', compares human life to a sea-journey and can be used as part of a 'Setting Off' activity.

Ovid
The *Metamorphoses* (Oxford: Oxford University Press, 1986) contains details of several characters from the *Odyssey*: Circe, the Cyclops, Odysseus himself (Ovid calls him 'Ulysses'), Scylla and Charybdis, as well as characters from Hades such as Tantalus and Sisyphus.

In the *Heroides* (London: Penguin 1990) Ovid includes a poem addressed by Penelope to her absent husband, Ulysses. There are also references to Ulysses and Circe in Ovid's *Love Poems* (Oxford: Oxford University Press, 1990) and *Erotic Poems* (London: Penguin, 1982). These poems are nearly 2000 years old.

Pound, Ezra
Canto I of *Selected Cantos* (London: Faber and Faber, 1967) contains a description of the descent of Odysseus to Hades.

Sackville, Margaret
The poem 'Romance' (*Collected Poems of Margaret, Lady Sackville,* London: Secker 1939) has a 'siren' like quality to the chorus and has been used in the Sirens episode.

Seferis, George
The *Collected Poems* (trans and ed by E. Keeley and P. Sherrard. London: Anvil Press, 1982) contains 'On a Line of Foreign Verse', which uses the voyage of Odysseus as its central image.

Shelley, Percy Bysshe
In the book of his collected poetry (*Poetical Works*, Oxford: Oxford University Press, 1970, trans 1819) can be found many poems that use the imagery of the sea, including 'Lines Written in the Euganean Hills', 'Adonais' and many more. Shelley also wrote many poems using figures from Greek mythology, including 'Hellas' and 'Prometheus Unbound' and translated the 'Cyclops' by Euripedes.

Spenser, Edmund
The epic poem *The Faerie Queene* (*Poetical Works*, Oxford: Oxford University Press, 1975) contains a description of Charybdis (II, XII, 3, 4–9[1]). There are more descriptions of Charybdis later on (II, XII, 6, 1–3; and II, XII, 20, 1–9), as well as descriptions of the Sirens (II, XII, 31, 1–9), The Wandering Rocks (II, XII, II, 3–9) and of Shipwreck (II, XII, 22, 1–4).

In his sonnet sequence *Amoretti*, there is a description of Penelope weaving at her loom and then unravelling her work at night (sonnet XXIII).

Tennyson, Alfred, Lord
Tennyson's Poetry (R.W. Hill (ed) New York: Norton, 1971) contains the poem 'Ulysses' and 'The Lotus Eaters'.

Tremain, Penelope
Under Helicon (Padstow: Tabb House, 1987) is a volume of poetry including several poems with references to sea-scapes and Greek locations. The lyrical title poem can be used in 'Setting Off' or 'Winding Down' activities.

Walcott, Derek
The Odyssey (London: Faber and Faber, 1993) is the author's stage play of the story. The language is poetic and extracts may be read as poetry.

His *Collected Poems* (London: Faber and Faber, 1992) contains many poems that use the imagery of the sea, for example, 'The Sea is History.'

Yeats, W.B.
The *Collected Poems* (London: MacMillan, 1973) contains several poems using imagery of the sea, for example 'Sailing to Byzantium', 'The Mermaid' and many more.

---

1   This notation reads for example Book II, Canto XII, Stanza 3, lines 4–9.

Keeping a Record During Sessions

Form 1. Individual Objectives

Name: **Date:**

1. Starting points

i. What meanings do you think the person can communicate? *Use the list in Figure 3.3 as a guide.*

eg. Requests

ii. How is meaning communicated? *Use the list in Figure 3.2 as a guide*

Making eye contact, vocalising.

Requests

Feelings

Comments

Turn-taking

Negatives

iii. What **sensory stimuli** are appropriate for the person?

Vision   Hearing   Touch   Smell

iv. What evidence does the person show of **pre-intentional** or **intentional** communication?

Pre-intentional

Reactive
Any consistent reactions to things or people?

Anticipatory
Any evidence of recognising what is about to happen?

Intentional

Intentional
Any evidence of deliberate communication with another person?

Reciprocal
Any evidence of awareness of and response to another person's reaction?

2. Where next? *Suggest one or two communicative behaviours that could be developed through the programme.*

3. Which games? *Suggest one or two games from the episodes you are planning to use which could be used to develop these communicative behaviours.*

4.i. What to look for *Decide what you want the person to do in response to the games.*

ii. *Decide what the staff role will be – how will you try to encourage this behaviour (e.g. prompting/demonstrating, pausing then prompting).*

5. First impressions. *Describe what the person actually did in response to the games you chose.*

6. Second thoughts? *Do you want to revise any of the goals, or change the games?*

YES/NO

IF SO, PUT YOUR IDEAS ON A NEW FORM.

Form 2: Individual Record

Name: _____   Date: _____

How meaning is communicated

What meanings are communicated	Body attitude	Using hands	Facial expression	Eye gaze	Vocalisation	Using objects	Gesture	Pointing	Use of pictures	Use of symbols	Use of manual signs	Use of speech	Level 1 2 3 4
Requests													
Feelings													
Comments													
Turn-Taking													
Negatives													

Level 1: Reactive   2. Anticipatory   3. Intentional   4. Reciprocal

Form 3: Group Record

Episode: Date:

Games
1.
3.
2.
4.

| Names | Target Behaviours
what you want to happen | Staff Role
how you encourage them to do it | Comments
what the person does |
|---|---|---|---|
| | | | |

References

Bates, E. (1976) *Language and Context: The Acquisition of Pragmatics.* New York: Academic Press.

Bates, E. Benigni, L., Bretherton, I., Camaioni, L. and Volterra, V. (1989) *The Emergence of Symbols: Cognition and Communication in Infancy.* New York: Academic Press.

Bolton, G. (1986) *Selected Writings on Drama in Education.* London, New York: Longman.

Bruner, J. (1963) *The Process of Education.* Cambridge, MA: Harvard University Press.

Bruner, J. (1983) *Child's Talk: Learning to use Language.* New York: Oxford University Press.

Bunting, B. (1994) *Collected Poems.* Oxford: Oxford University Press.

Campbell, C.H. and Wilcox, M.J. (1986) Communicative effectiveness of movement patterns used by non-vocal children with severe handicaps. Stockholm, Sweden. *Paper presented at the Fourth International Conference of the International Society for Augmentative and Alternative Communication, Cardiff, Wales.*

Coupe, J. and Goldbart, J. (1987) *Communication Before Speech.* London: Croom Helm.

Department of Education (1995) *Key Stahes 1 and 2 of the National Curriculum.* London: HMSO.

Dante (1961) *The Divine Comedy. 1: The Inferno* (trans J.D. Sinclair). Oxford: Oxford University Press.

Dunst, C. and Lowe, L. (1986) From reflex to symbol: describing, explaining and fostering communicative competence. *Augmentative and Alternative Communication 2,* 11–18.

Faforgue, J. (1985) *Moral Tales* (trans W.J. Smith). London: Picador.

Goldbart, J. (1994) Opening the communication curriculum to students with PMLDs. In J. Ward (ed) *Educating Children with Profound and Multiple Learning Difficulties.* David Fulton: London.

Graves, R. (1981) *The Greek Myths: 2.* London: Pelican.

Inner London Education Authority Consortium (1984) *Galaxies.* London: Inner London Education Authority Consortium.

Lock, A. (1978) *Action, Gesture and Symbol: The Emergence of Language.* New York: Academic Press.

McLean, J. and Snyder-McLean, L. (1988) Application of pragmatics to severely mentally retarded children and youth. In R.L. Schiefelbusch and L.L. Lloyd (eds) *Language Perspectives: Acquisition, Retardation and Intervention* (2nd edition, pp.255–288). Austin, TX: ProED.

Mount, H. (1995) 'Art, drama and music.' In J. Hogg and J. Cavet (eds) *Making Leisure Provision for People with Profound Learning and Multiple Disabilities.* London: Chapman and Hall.

Neelands, J. (1992) *Learning Through Imagined Experience.* London: Hodder and Stoughton.

Nind, M. and Hewett, D. (1994) *Access to Communication.* London: David Fulton.

Park, K. (1991) A communication course for adults with profound intellectual disability and physical disabilities: Part 1. *Mental Handicap 19,* 4, 165–169.

Park, K. (1992) Developing the environment: Part 2 (unpublished).

Park, K., Robinson, B. and Williams, C. (1989) *Communication as Curriculum.* London: SENJIT (Special Needs Joint Initiative for Training)/London University Institute of Education.

Robinson, T. and Curtis, R. (1986) *Odysseus, the Greatest Hero of Them All.* London: BBC/Knight.

Rowland, C. and Schweigert, P. (1989) Tangible symbols: symbolic communication for individuals with multisensory impairments. *Augmentative and Alternative Communication 5,* 226–234.

Rubens, B. and Taplin, O. (1989) *An Odyssey Around Odysseus.* London: BBC Books.

Siegel-Causey, E. and Guess, D. (1989) *Enhancing Nonsymbolic Communication Interaction among Learners with Severe Disabilities.* Baltimore: Paul H. Brookes Publishing.

Sperber, D. and Wilson, D. (1986) *Relevance: Communication and Cognition.* Oxford: Blackwell.

Sternberg, L. Ehren, B., Leferts, L. and Eloranta, R. (1988) Assessing non-linguistic communication skills of students with severe or profound handicaps: towards a research agenda. *Journal of Childhood Communication Disorders 11,* 275–286.

Sternberg, L. and Owens, A. (1985) Establishing pre-language signalling behaviour with profoundly mentally handicapped students: A preliminary investigation. *Journal of Mental Deficiency Research 29,* 81–93.

Vygotsky (1976) 'Play and its role in the mental development of the child.' In J.S. Bruner, A. Jolly and K. Sylva (eds) *Play: Its Role in Development and Evolution.* Harmondsworth: Penguin Education.

Vygotsky (1978) *Mind in Society.* Cambridge, MA: Harvard University Press.

Ware, J. (1989) Designing appropriate environments for people with PMLD. In W. Fraser (ed) *Key Issues in Mental Retardation Research.* London: Methuen.

Ware, J. (1994) Using interaction in the education of pupils with PMLDs (i) Creating contingency-sensitive environments. In J. Ware (ed) *Educating Children with Profound and Multiple Learning Difficulties.* London: David Fulton.

Webb, E. (1992) *Literature in Education.* London: Falmer Press.

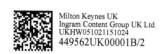

Milton Keynes UK
Ingram Content Group UK Ltd.
UKHW051021151024
449562UK00001B/2

9 781853 023156